The
ABCs
of
Breastfeeding

The
ABCs
of
Breastfeeding

Everything a Mom Needs to Know
for a Happy Nursing Experience

Stacey H. Rubin, M.N., APRN, IBCLC

AMACOM
New York • Atlanta • Brussels • Chicago
Mexico City • San Francisco • Shanghai • Tokyo • Toronto • Washington, D.C.

Special discounts on bulk quantities of AMACOM books are
available to corporations, professional associations, and other
organizations. For details, contact Special Sales Department,
AMACOM, a division of American Management Association,
1601 Broadway, New York, NY 10019.
Tel.: 212-903-8316.   Fax: 212-903-8083.
Web Site: www.amacombooks.org

All examples were composite in nature. Furthermore, all names and identifying details have
been changed to protect my clients' privacy. Every effort has been made to ensure that the
information contained in this book is complete and accurate. However, neither the publisher
nor the author is engaged in rendering professional advice or services to the individual reader.
The ideas, procedures, and suggestions contained in this book are not intended as a substitute
for consulting your health-care provider. All matters regarding the health of you and your baby
require medical supervision. Neither the publisher nor the author shall be liable or responsible
for any loss or damage allegedly arising from any information or suggestions in this book.

Various names used by companies to distinguish their software and other products can be
claimed as trademarks. AMACOM uses such names throughout this book for editorial
purposes only, with no intention of trademark violation. All such software or product
names are in initial capital letters or ALL CAPITAL letters. Individual companies
should be contacted for complete information regarding trademarks and registration.

Library of Congress Cataloging-in-Publication Data

Rubin, Stacey H.
    The ABCs of breastfeeding : everything a mom needs to know for
a happy nursing experience / Stacey H. Rubin.
        p.   cm.
    Includes bibliographical references and index.
    ISBN 978-0-8144-8057-1 (pbk.)
    1. Breastfeeding.   I. Title.

RJ216.R835 2008
649'.33—dc22
                            2007048160

Printing number

10   9   8   7   6   5   4   3   2   1

This book is dedicated to the mothers and babies

who have been my clients.

Contents

Contents

✿

Phase II
Beginning to Breastfeed Your Baby ▪ 81

✿

Phase III
Continuing to Breastfeed Comfortably into the Future ▪ 147

◦ᴿ

Phase IV
Developing Your Own Happy Ending ■ 201

Preface

I t seems unlikely that I would have grown to care so passionately about babies and breastfeeding. After all, I was not breastfed, and by three years of age, I was adept at helping my newly divorced overworked mother formula feed my younger twin sisters. While my mother tended to one of my sisters, I would hold a bottle for the other baby as she sat propped in an infant seat. This way, my mother could have both babies fed simultaneously. In my eyes, babies were born to bottle-feed.

I will never forget the first time I saw a mother breastfeed her baby. I was a twenty-two-year-old senior nursing student rotating through the labor and delivery ward of a busy hospital in downtown Philadelphia. I stood mesmerized as a mother gave birth to her fourth child in a drafty delivery room. Minutes later, oblivious to the chaos of hospital staff rushing in and out of the room, mother and baby found each other, and the naked baby girl began to nurse as if she were born in that moment for just that purpose.

A year later, I was a brand-new lieutenant stationed in California, three thousand miles away from familiar Philadelphia. Army nurses are expected to be versatile, caring for soldiers with broken bones in the emergency room one day and psychiatric patients with broken minds the next day. I wasn't surprised when without warning I was assigned baby duty in the hospital nursery. I knew next to nothing about babies and even less about breastfeeding, and yet, I was suddenly responsible for teaching new mothers to breastfeed their newborns. I watched helplessly as most mothers met with failure and left the hospital feeding their babies formula that military families couldn't afford. I wondered why breastfeeding was so difficult when it had been so effortless for that mother I had seen when I was a student.

Four years later, I reentered the civilian world and enrolled in a Florida graduate school. The advanced practice nursing program required long clinical hours in the neonatal intensive care unit, where I learned to manage the medical care of the smallest and sickest babies. Incredibly, not a single hour of this rigorous program was devoted to the art and science of bringing a mother and baby together to breastfeed.

After I relocated to Connecticut and made a career caring for the babies of strangers, my husband, Timothy, and I became parents to Miriam. I began to breastfeed. It wasn't always easy. Miriam was born earlier than expected and was slow to gain weight. Just after Miriam's second birthday, our son Max was born at home with a midwife in attendance. Max was born directly into my arms and breastfed immediately, like that baby girl I had seen nearly fifteen years ago when I was new to all of this.

Daily life with two young children was demanding—no more spur-of-the-moment vacations, elaborately prepared meals, or sleeping late on weekends. Our once spotless living room now looked like a playroom. Besides the outward changes, motherhood was changing me on the inside as well. I was becoming more patient, less structured, and more tolerant of ambiguity. Even my sense of time was becoming less militaristic. It seemed that the minutes of one day drifted into the next week. I remember bringing Miriam to breast one snowy New England afternoon;

when we finished that feeding, winter had morphed into spring, and the lawn was dotted with purple crocuses.

After breastfeeding Miriam and Max, I yearned to bring mothers and babies together rather than separate them with hospital procedures. Out of that desire, I founded my private practice, and I began visiting mothers in their homes throughout Connecticut. This book reflects what I have discovered about mothers, babies, and breastfeeding over the years. My clients have been my best teachers, and I tell their stories in the pages of this text. My clients are real moms just like you, and chances are you will identify with their struggles and applaud their triumphs. Most of all, I hope that you are able to apply the step-by-step advice in each chapter to your unique situation, and that you use my advice to make your breastfeeding experience a happy one. Since most breastfeeding problems can be avoided, I stress steps that you can take to avert problems before they arise. Because breastfeeding is a science as well as an art, whenever possible, I have included evidence-based citations in the manuscript to support my advice.

As you read this book, my hope is that you will become the recipient of breastfeeding's greatest gifts. Regardless of how long you breastfeed your baby or how much milk you produce, breastfeeding is an experience like no other. Learning to trust the process instead of analyzing it is a leap of faith for most mothers. That's exactly how it was for me. When I became a breastfeeding mother, I had no idea that breastfeeding would shift the direction of my life. As with all journeys, it has been the experience of traveling rather than the destination that has left me forever transformed.

Back then, I had been trained to trust formula and had little understanding of the biology of mother's milk. I knew only that it was made close to my heart, infused with living cells, and dispensed at the temperature of life. Having had their fill of breast milk, both of my babies have blossomed into busy children, but I imagine that they can still taste the milk of their mother's eternal love.

Acknowledgments

First and foremost, I would like to thank my husband, Timothy J. Holsbeke, for his constant support as well as for typing and formatting the entire manuscript into the computer at night after working all day. Thank you to my children, Miriam and Max, for giving me real life lessons in birth and breastfeeding. I want to thank my agent, Patricia Snell, and my editor, Ellen Kadin; without a doubt, both of you are the best in the business. I want to thank and acknowledge the entire NICU staff of Connecticut Children's Medical Center, especially the extraordinary group of neonatal nurse practitioners, physician assistants, professional nurses, lactation consultants, respiratory therapists, and neonatalogists. This unit performs miracles on a daily basis under the compassionate leadership of Victor Herson. Thank you to the La Leche League and its leaders for their unwavering commitment to breastfeeding mothers. Thank you to Christina Smillie and Kathie Marinelli for encouraging me to become a lactation consultant. Thank you to Pete Considine, Jacqueline Newhouse, and Ben Silberman for working on the proposal. Thank you to Linda Kaczmarczyk for your indispensable research assistance.

Thank you to Nancy Kozak for being an excellent doula and to Nan Kyer for being an excellent lactation consultant. Thank you to Wendolyn Hill for the illustrations in this book. Thank you to Joe Moreno for being a wonderful stylist and confidant throughout the years. Thank you to Lisa Slot for your friendship, humor, and support. I am indebted to Nancy Aronie for providing me with inspiration. A big thank-you to the entire staff of the Bishop's Corner Starbucks for all of the warm smiles and hot coffee while I worked. Finally, I want to thank my two beautiful yoga teachers, John Dorsey and Karen Wagner.

Phase I

Things to Consider Before Birth

During my years as a neonatal nurse practitioner and lactation consultant, I have worked with hundreds of new parents and their babies, and have come to realize that the breastfeeding process begins before birth. Whether you are a new or experienced mother, the conscious and unconscious choices you make as your pregnancy progresses will have a tremendous impact on your future as a breastfeeding mother. From the beginning, your body in its infinite wisdom prepares to breastfeed. Addressing six important issues during this time before birth will give you the opportunity to create a positive beginning to your breastfeeding experience.

CHAPTER ONE

Thinking with a Breastfeeding Mindset

"I'll try breastfeeding, but I don't think
that it is going to work."
—AMY

my is preparing for the birth of her first child. She and her
husband have taken a childbirth education class and a breastfeeding class and are in the process of reading two breastfeeding books. Despite all that she has learned, Amy remains
doubtful about the prospect of breastfeeding the daughter she is expecting. All of Amy's knowledge about breastfeeding can't compete with her
defeatist attitude. Any problem that arises as she adjusts to her new baby
will derail the breastfeeding process and prevent her from finding a workable solution to whatever difficulty she may have. For breastfeeding to
work after her baby is born, Amy must develop a positive attitude during
pregnancy. A positive attitude is not an accident. As you will learn in this
chapter, you are the gardener of your psyche; only you can till the soil of
your mind and cultivate a positive breastfeeding mindset.

DOES MY ATTITUDE ABOUT BREASTFEEDING REALLY MATTER?

During pregnancy, you are like an athlete in training. Your body is performing the Herculean task of growing a baby. While your body gets ready for motherhood, you—like the coach of a winning team—have the unique opportunity to prepare your mind for breastfeeding success. All coaches train their players to be strong and fast on the field; however, the coach of a winning team is able to do something extra that consistently leads his or her team to victory. The coach of a winning team instills a winning attitude in each player. Coaches understand that games are won or lost in the minds of their players. Players with a positive attitude play to win, whereas players full of self-doubt sabotage the team. On game day, all the hours of grueling physical training will be lost on an athlete who approaches the playing field lacking self-confidence. The seasoned successful coach prepares the team's minds as well as their muscles.

Like a competitive athlete psyching out an opponent before the start of the game, breastfeeding begins in a mother's psyche before her baby is born. Whether or not you are aware of it, your conscious and subconscious attitude about breastfeeding will profoundly affect your future breastfeeding relationship with your baby. As your pregnancy progresses, you may be preoccupied with work, child care, or shopping for your new baby. Even though you are busy, set aside a moment to explore your personal attitude about breastfeeding. A mother's attitude sets the tone for her entire breastfeeding experience.

Chances are, like Amy, you have developed some negative perceptions about breastfeeding. Mothers develop these perceptions for a variety of reasons including formula company advertising, their body image, and difficulties with breastfeeding in the past. Understanding how these factors shape your view of breastfeeding will allow you to recognize your personal feelings about breastfeeding before your baby is born.

HOW DOES FORMULA MARKETING AFFECT
MY VIEW OF BREASTFEEDING?

Because advertising portrays formula feeding as the normal way to nourish a baby, it is one of the most powerful influences against breastfeeding in our society. Television commercials show smiling mothers who happily feed bottles of formula to their babies. The latest trend in advertising is to hire a celebrity mom to endorse a formula that she supposedly feeds her baby. Celebrity association with anything, whether it's perfume or infant formula, makes the product seem chic and sophisticated. In addition, parenting magazines also advertise formula, bottles, and pacifiers. I recently saw a magazine advertisement picturing an infant and a calf sitting side by side together in a double stroller. The advertisement was for a newfangled bottle claiming to keep a baby's feeding as fresh as if it had just come from a cow. Many formulas claim their artificial ingredients are "formulated" like breast milk, and bottles claim to be shaped like a human nipple. Although ridiculous, these ads, coupled with sophisticated marketing techniques that operate on a psychological level, persuade millions of mothers that formula is convenient, risk-free, and comparable to human milk. Regardless of what advertisements tell you, the truth is that breast milk is uniquely suited to meet your baby's needs, and your milk cannot be duplicated in a factory.

Unfortunately, formula advertising is impossible to escape. Ready-to-feed bottles of formula are directly marketed to parents by mail.[1] In nearly every client's home that I visit, I can't help but notice a formula sample pack sitting innocuously on the kitchen counter. With formula samples so readily available, it becomes easy for mothers to succumb to bottle-feeding in a moment of doubt. Receiving a formula sample can undermine a mother's confidence even when breastfeeding is progressing well.

My client, Sheila, is a twenty-year-old mother who has been breastfeeding her son, Cameron, since birth. Cameron is now a healthy nine-month-old and has never had formula. I was surprised when Sheila called me wondering whether Cameron needed to start formula at nine months of age. Sheila had just received a formula sample supposedly designed for older babies. I assured Sheila that her breast milk was still perfectly formulated for Cameron and discouraged her from feeding her son the artificial food.

Formula manufacturers, or pharmaceutical companies, provide pediatric offices and most hospitals with cases of free formula to distribute to their patients. By accepting and distributing formula, doctors and nurses reinforce the idea that formula feeding is the normal option and undermine any positive ideas new mothers have in deciding to breastfeed their babies.

Isabel, as a single mother, had her hands full with healthy twin boys. When I met with Isabel, she had a tremendous milk supply and her sons breastfed easily. However, Isabel was in the habit of formula feeding the twins throughout the day. She continued to feed the twins bottles because the hospital had given them formula after they were born and had sent her home with several boxes of the stuff. As a result of this pervasive advertising, Isabel, like many mothers, believed that formula was just as healthy as breast milk.

Formula samples cleverly disguised as hospital gift bags and distributed to new mothers by nurses can undermine a new mother's breastfeeding relationship by reducing the likelihood that she will exclusively breastfeed her newborn.[2] Some hospitals designated as Baby-Friendly have stopped the practice of routinely distributing formula samples to new mothers and no longer accept free formula from the pharmaceutical companies.

WHY IS BREAST MILK BETTER THAN FORMULA?

What formula advertising won't tell you is that there is no substitute for human milk. Human milk is a living food made specifically for the unique needs of human babies. The best scientists in the world cannot re-create its more than two hundred components in a laboratory. Unlike the artificial ingredients in formula, which never change, your breast milk will evolve to meet the specific needs of your growing baby. This is true whether you breastfeed for one week or one year.

To begin with, nature designed your newborn's first feeding of colostrum to be small in volume and high in value. Yellow or golden in color, colostrum, or early breast milk, is in your breasts when your baby is born. The components of colostrum are uniquely concentrated to both nourish and protect a brand-new baby. Compared to more mature breast milk, colostrum is higher in cholesterol, protein, and minerals like sodium and magnesium.[3] Colostrum also contains high levels of immunoglobulin "A," which protects your baby's developing gastrointestinal tract from foreign germs and allergens.[4] Even one exposure to formula at this critical time can upset this delicate balance in your baby's intestines.[5]

As the first days of motherhood pass, your colostrum gradually becomes white in color. This transitional milk has high concentrations of living white cells called macrophages that continue the work of providing immunological protection to your newborn. Over the next few days, the ratio of proteins, fats, vitamins, and minerals continues to shift, resulting in perfectly balanced mature breast milk.[6] Mature breast milk is smart food. Complex fats and proteins promote your baby's rapidly developing brain. Research has demonstrated that children who have been breastfed have higher intelligence than their formula-fed schoolmates.[7] When a mother and baby eventually begin the weaning process and the total volume of a mother's milk is reduced, the living cells in breast milk faithfully continue to protect a baby from illness.

CAN I BREASTFEED IF MY BABY IS BORN EARLY?

Like a commissioned piece of art, breast milk can never be replicated. Each mother's milk is designed to meet the unique needs of her baby; no two samples of breast milk are exactly alike. For instance, the pumped breast milk sampled from Joyce, the mother of a preterm infant born ten weeks early and being cared for in the neonatal intensive care unit, contains higher concentrations of fat, protein, immunoglobulin, and certain minerals than the milk from the mother of a baby born at full term.[8] When analyzed, the fats within Joyce's preterm breast milk differ significantly from those found in full-term breast milk. Joyce's milk is well suited for her premature son's underdeveloped stomach and intestine. In fact, providing pumped milk for her hospitalized son will speed his recovery and lower the likelihood of him developing complications such as a life-threatening infection.[9]

New research suggests just how individualized breast milk may be. The specific sequence of amino acids that join to form the complex proteins in breast milk may be unique to each mother, like the swirls of her fingerprint.[10] On a daily basis, the volume of breast milk adjusts to accommodate the changes in a baby's appetite. A mother's appetite may also vary, and her food preferences are reflected in the taste of her breast milk.[11] Always sweetened by the milk-sugar lactose, breast milk will be infused with different flavors depending on a mother's daily diet.

ARE MY BREASTS THE RIGHT SIZE AND SHAPE FOR BREASTFEEDING?

Understanding that breastfeeding provides your baby with unparalleled health advantages may not be enough to overcome all the negative messages related to breastfeeding that abound in our society. In addition to presenting bottle-feeding as the norm, the media fosters an unrealistic image of the female body in this country. This is important to consider as a woman's feelings about her breasts can undermine her confidence in her natural ability to breastfeed. Most women's bodies differ from the ideal female figure portrayed on television and in magazines. The national obsession for perfectly shaped breasts is evident in the high number of cosmetic breast surgeries performed in this country. As a result, many mothers are now dealing with the challenges of breastfeeding a baby following breast augmentation or breast reduction surgery.

What many women don't realize is that the breasts they were born with will work for the purpose for which they were intended. Almost any breast and nipple works to feed a baby. Unfortunately, most women wrongly assume that their breastfeeding problems are caused by faulty anatomy. Upon examination, I usually find that all these mothers who are worried about their anatomy have normal breasts and are able to breastfeed.

The lactating breast is a dynamic organ. Breasts and nipples undergo changes during pregnancy and continue to evolve during lactation. Differences between the left and right breasts are common since our bodies are not completely symmetrical. For instance, most women are surprised to learn that it is normal for one breast to produce more milk than the other.[12] Without this knowledge, women may have a hard time believing that their bodies are functioning normally and begin to doubt their body's natural ability to breastfeed. Each mother-baby pair is unique; have faith that your baby will be a perfect match for the size and shape of the breasts and nipples you were born with.

LACK OF SUCCESS BREASTFEEDING YOUR FIRST BABY DOESN'T MEAN YOU CAN'T WITH YOUR SECOND

Perhaps the most powerful factor that shapes a mother's perception about breastfeeding is her personal history and experience with breastfeeding. A previous inability to breastfeed may leave a mother with painful memories. Afraid of experiencing the same difficulty, she may lack the self-confidence to breastfeed a subsequent baby. Marla was a client who had been unsuccessful breastfeeding her first daughter and wanted to try again with the daughter she was expecting. During our prenatal consultation, Marla shared with me a lengthy family history of breastfeeding woes beginning with her mother, aunt, sisters, and ending with her. We talked for quite a while about what steps she could take that would lead to breastfeeding success, but Marla seemed unconvinced that her future could be better than her past. After giving birth, she called me from the hospital to cancel our next appointment because she had decided not to breastfeed after all.

IF MY MOTHER COULDN'T BREASTFEED, WILL I HAVE THE SAME PROBLEMS?

Mothers often tell me that they are ambivalent about their ability to breastfeed because no one in their family has successfully breastfed. Lacking a positive example, a new mother may believe that breastfeeding will never work for her. I tell mothers that even if no woman in their immediate family has successfully breastfed, it's inevitable that somewhere in the branches of the family tree, a woman had an abundant milk flow and breastfed one of their relatives. Now it is your turn to reclaim that breastfeeding tradition for the next generation.

Don't allow your past breastfeeding difficulty to spoil a future breastfeeding relationship. In order to move forward, you must first acknowledge any past disappointment with breastfeeding. Look back with curiosity, not blame, to see what you might have done differently and what you can change in the future. Not only is each baby a unique individual, but your body changes with each new pregnancy. Recognize this as a new chance to make breastfeeding work for you. That is exactly what my client Marissa did. Marissa called me after her second child, Jacob, was born. During our consultation, Marissa told me that she had given up on breastfeeding her first son shortly after he was born. This time Marissa had an air of determination about her. She wanted to find a workable solution to the difficulty she faced. Eventually, breastfeeding became easier for Marissa and last I heard, she was still breastfeeding Jacob.

WHAT IS THE MOST EFFECTIVE BREASTFEEDING MINDSET?

Over the years, I've worked with many different types of clients: from professors to artists; from doctors to stay-at-home mothers—all of whom strongly desired a breastfeeding relationship with their babies. Their breast-feeding problems were as varied as their careers and personalities, and the clients that went on to have the most satisfying breastfeeding relationships with their babies all shared what I call a *positive breastfeeding mindset*. A positive breastfeeding mindset is a deeply felt belief that breastfeeding will work, and that with a little help, mother and baby can learn to breast-feed. This attitude is a mother's best defense against formula company advertising, a negative body image, and past breastfeeding difficulties. Mothers with a positive breastfeeding mindset make breastfeeding a priority and take deliberate steps to make it work. When an obstacle arises in their breastfeeding relationship, a mother with a positive breastfeeding mindset seeks qualified assistance. (If you're reading this book, you've already taken a good step!) Having a positive attitude enables a mother to accept the help she needs and persevere until her problem is solved.

My client Kate personifies this mindset. Kate gave birth to her first child, William, a week after relocating to a new area. When I went to visit them, their apartment was full of unpacked boxes. Kate had been told by several doctors that breastfeeding would be difficult because her breasts were different sizes. Her doctors doubted that Kate's unequal breasts could produce enough milk. Kate and William did have a rocky start. Following a complicated birth, William spent time in the hospital nursery, where he was fed formula. Once home from the hospital, breastfeeding continued to be a challenge. Separated from family, unsure of her body, and with a bag full of formula samples, Kate could have given up on breastfeeding altogether. When Kate and I met for our consultation, she told me that with the right help and enough time she knew that breastfeeding would work. Kate and William followed a step-by-step plan, and over the course of a few weeks Kate found that breastfeeding became easier. William is now three months old and continues to breastfeed. I believe that Kate's positive attitude about breastfeeding enabled her to persevere through a difficult start.

If you are pregnant and have the desire to breastfeed your baby, now is the time to face any negative thoughts or feelings you may have about breastfeeding. Perhaps you and your siblings were formula fed, and you have grown up without a breastfeeding example. You may have believed the advertising that formula is just as healthy as breast milk. Maybe you are ambivalent about using your breasts for their natural purpose of feeding your baby. If you don't already have a positive breastfeeding mindset, you can still create one.

HOW DOES ONE DEVELOP A POSITIVE BREASTFEEDING MINDSET?

When it comes to breastfeeding, you can coach your mind into a winning attitude. As you take the necessary steps to prepare your mindset, your body will do the rest. From the beginning of pregnancy, your body assumes that you will breastfeed, so it prepares colostrum for your baby's first meal. Over the length of pregnancy, milk ducts in your breasts will proliferate, causing your breasts to grow in size. While you focus on preparing your mindset, trust that your body is doing its job and will be ready to breastfeed. You can take the first step toward a positive breastfeeding mindset by creating a breastfeeding affirmation and repeating it daily. An affirmation is a positive statement that has personal meaning. For example, near the end of her pregnancy, Clara feared she would not produce an abundant milk supply after her baby was born. She created the following affirmation to change her mindset: "When my baby is born, my body will make plenty of milk." Eventually, your affirmation will take hold in your subconscious mind and you will gain self-confidence in your ability to breastfeed.

Peggy's breastfeeding success is a testament to the power of a positive breastfeeding mindset. I met Peggy and her husband, Todd, when they were expecting their first child, and I was teaching the breastfeeding segment of a childbirth education class. On this particular evening Maggie, the childbirth instructor, asked me to shorten my presentation because she had a lot of material left to cover with her students before the series ended.

Even though I was disappointed that these soon-to-be parents wouldn't be getting the benefit of a complete breastfeeding class, I agreed to teach an abbreviated class. Rather than lecture about the mechanics of breast-feeding, I dedicated most of the short class to the importance of develop-ing a positive breastfeeding mindset during pregnancy. I remember Peggy, seated in the front row, took plenty of notes as we reviewed examples of breastfeeding affirmations. Several weeks later, I ran into Peggy, Todd, and their brand-new baby, Henry. Peggy was beaming with pride when she told me that she was breastfeeding Henry. Peggy explained that before our breastfeeding class, she had been very nervous about breastfeeding. After-ward, she faithfully practiced the breastfeeding affirmations that she had learned, and without any further formal training, she was able to confi-dently breastfeed Henry.

HOW TO CREATE YOUR OWN
BREASTFEEDING AFFIRMATION

The first step in developing a breastfeeding affirmation is to identify a neg-ative feeling about breastfeeding or your body's ability to nurture your baby. Next, write down the negative statement and change it into a positive one. For the affirmation to be effective, the statement must be personal, so use terms like "my breast" and "my baby." Once you have identified at least one personal breastfeeding affirmation, write it down and place it where you will repeatedly see it. Repeat your affirmation out loud in the car and in the shower. Look in the mirror and say the affirmation every day. Soon the affirmation will take hold and have a positive effect on your future breastfeeding relationship.

Suggested affirmations for a positive breastfeeding mindset

My breasts are the perfect size for my baby.
My breasts will fill with abundant milk for my baby.

My baby and I will find the perfect fit for breastfeeding.

When my baby is born, I will be ready to breastfeed.

My milk is the best way for me to nourish my baby.

If I encounter breastfeeding difficulty, someone will help me.

WHAT ELSE CAN I DO TO DEVELOP A POSITIVE BREASTFEEDING MINDSET?

Breastfeeding affirmations will retrain how you think about breastfeeding. Visualization exercises can further strengthen your positive breastfeeding mindset. We tend to live out what it is we imagine for ourselves. By filling your mind with positive images of breastfeeding, you create a powerful self-fulfilling prophecy. The following visualization exercise is designed to fill your mind with an enjoyable stress-free picture of breastfeeding. The exercise works best if a partner reads the visualization to you as you relax with your eyes closed. If possible, find a pregnant friend to share this exercise with you. You may wish to create your own personal visualization by conjuring up an image of yourself joyfully breastfeeding your newborn. Don't worry about the logistical details of breastfeeding; just allow your mind's eye to make it happen. Be alert for any negative thoughts that arise during these exercises, so you can turn those thoughts into positive affirmations. Continue to strengthen your positive breastfeeding mindset until your baby is born.

Visualization for a positive breastfeeding mindset

Sit comfortably, breathe deeply, and close your eyes.

Inhale and exhale fully at a comfortable pace.

Sit up straight, making plenty of room for your baby to breathe with you.

Place your hands on your pregnant abdomen and hug your baby from the outside.

Assure your baby that he or she is safe and loved inside of you.

Envision picking up your baby after birth.

Hold your baby close to your chest so that your baby can begin to breastfeed.

Your baby is breastfeeding perfectly.

Take a few more deep breaths.

End your visualization by hugging your baby from outside of your body, and repeat your affirmation for breastfeeding success.

SUMMARY OF BREASTFEEDING ABCs

As you have learned, your internal view of breastfeeding affects your future success. A positive breastfeeding mindset will enable you to recognize and overcome obstacles should they arise in your breastfeeding relationship. As you prepare for your journey into motherhood, make breastfeeding a priority by taking the time to create a positive mindset. If you have negative thoughts and feelings about breastfeeding, practicing affirmations and visualizations will enable you to create a more positive mindset. Thinking like a breastfeeding mother before the time to breastfeed comes is the first step that will lead you to a satisfying breastfeeding relationship with your baby.

A. ATTITUDE

Examine your personal attitudes about breastfeeding. Negative thoughts and feelings about it will hinder your future breastfeeding relationship with your baby. Many factors influence a woman's perceptions about breastfeeding. More often than not, the media portrays breastfeeding as difficult and time consuming; formula companies promote bottle-feeding as the normal way to feed a baby, and experienced mothers may be negatively affected by the memory of past breastfeeding difficulty. Gaining awareness of your feelings will allow you to take steps to change your negative thoughts and approach breastfeeding with a positive mindset.

B. BODY

Trust your body. Your body assumes that you will breastfeed your newborn baby. As your baby develops during pregnancy, your breasts undergo changes in preparation for breastfeeding. Cells inside your breasts begin to produce colostrum for your baby's first meal. Colostrum is yellow or golden color, thick, and usually small in volume. In addition to protecting your newborn from infection, colostrum prepares your baby's stomach and intestines for higher volumes of mature breast milk. Even if your baby is born earlier than expected, your body will produce colostrum and breast milk. Pregnancy and birth prepare your body in every way to breastfeed your baby.

C. CREATION

Create a positive breastfeeding mindset. Learn how to reframe your mind for breastfeeding success. If you have negative thoughts and feelings, now is the time to alter your thinking. In addition to the breastfeeding affirmations included in this chapter, feel free to develop your own personal breastfeeding affirmations. To do this, first recognize any negative thoughts or feelings you may harbor about breastfeeding. Next, change that thought or feeling into a positive, personal statement about breastfeeding. Write your affirmation down and place it where you will see it. Affirmations along with visualization serve to build a positive breastfeeding mindset and are your first step toward learning to breastfeed successfully.

CHAPTER TWO

Finding a Breastfeeding-Friendly Doctor

"Everyone is telling me something different,
and I don't know what to believe."
—KATIE

ecently, I visited Katie, a first-time mother at forty years old,
who was determined to breastfeed her twin girls, Audrey and
Elaine. During our consultation, Audrey and Elaine breastfed
beautifully, and I recommended a plan that combined breastfeeding and pumping milk for the twins. Audrey and Elaine were healthy
and thriving on their mother's abundant milk supply. Several days after our
consult, Katie called confused and upset following a visit with the twins'
pediatrician. The pediatrician instructed her to limit the babies to a few
minutes of breastfeeding and feed them bottles of formula according to his
prescribed schedule. Instead of commending the excellent work Katie was
doing for her babies, he carried a case of formula to her husband's car in
the parking lot. His advice combined with the formula samples demor-
alized this mother's breastfeeding efforts.

Katie chose her pediatrician because his practice was conveniently
close to her husband's office. Had Katie considered other criteria besides
geography, she may have chosen a different pediatrician and saved her
breastfeeding relationship with the twins. Like Katie, many busy parents

17

choose a doctor for themselves and their baby based on the location of the office. If this is your only criterion, you may be satisfied with your choice. However, if you plan to use your pediatrician as a breastfeeding resource, you may be disappointed. Almost all health-care professionals say that "breastfeeding is best." I remind my clients that their goal is to find a doctor who sincerely *means* it! A breastfeeding-friendly pediatrician should be able to provide accurate, supportive advice and be willing to refer complex breastfeeding problems to a certified lactation consultant.

ARE DOCTORS TRAINED TO SUPPORT BREASTFEEDING?

Unfortunately, doctors receive little or no education about breastfeeding in medical school.[1] After graduating from medical school, doctors work as residents in a hospital for several years where their only exposure to breastfeeding mothers and babies may come from working with a lactation consultant during their newborn nursery rotation. Unless the hospital where a new doctor trains is designated as Baby-Friendly by the World Health Organization (WHO), the new doctor—along with the rest of the hospital staff—will be subjected to formula advertising including biased educational materials written by the same pharmaceutical companies that manufacture infant formula. All of this reinforces the supposed normalcy of formula feeding for the young doctor. After years of training, the end result is a cadre of enthusiastic new pediatricians whose only reference for normal newborn feeding behavior is a baby who eats measured amounts of a prescribed formula at scheduled intervals from a bottle.

In an effort to increase physician support of breastfeeding, the American Academy of Pediatrics (AAP) issued a policy statement recommending that all pediatricians promote, protect, and support breastfeeding.[2] The new statement issued in the winter of 2005 recognized the unparalleled health benefits that breastfeeding provides to mothers and babies. (The health benefits that breastfeeding provides to *mothers* is discussed later in this chapter.) This new policy delineates steps that pediatricians can take in their private offices to encourage mothers to exclusively breastfeed their babies for six months. Among other things, the AAP discourages the display of formula advertising and the distribution of formula packs to new mothers. In other words, a pediatrician who practices according to the AAP policy statement is a breastfeeding ally.

DOES IT MATTER IF MY OBSTETRICIAN SUPPORTS BREASTFEEDING?

As we learned in Chapter One, a positive breastfeeding mindset is your first step toward future breastfeeding success. Receiving prenatal care from an obstetrician or midwife who is a breastfeeding ally can serve to reinforce your positive breastfeeding mindset. During office visits, a breastfeeding ally will take the time to explain how breastfeeding your baby can significantly improve *your* overall health. One of my clients admitted she had been "on the fence" as to whether to breastfeed her baby until she was in the delivery room and her obstetrician convinced her to breastfeed.

The benefits of breastfeeding begin right after your baby is born. For example, as you breastfeed your baby, the hormone oxytocin activates your milk flow and helps your uterus regain its tone after birth. This process prevents excessive bleeding as you recover from childbirth. Research has also shown that women who breastfeed have a reduced risk of developing breast cancer, ovarian cancer, and urinary tract infections.[3] Since making a full supply of breast milk for one baby requires about 500 extra calories a day, mothers who breastfeed tend to lose weight gained during pregnancy faster than mothers who do not breastfeed.[4] After a mother stops breastfeeding, her bones re-mineralize, or become stronger, thus decreasing the likelihood that she will develop osteoporosis in later life.[5]

DOES IT MATTER IF MY PEDIATRICIAN SUPPORTS BREASTFEEDING?

I was happy to receive a phone call one Friday afternoon from a local pediatrician; I was not acquainted with this doctor, but after listening to her concerns, I knew she was a breastfeeding ally. She was worried about a young mother whose ten-day-old breastfed baby had lost weight. As far as she could tell from her office exam, this first-time mother was making a lot of milk and the baby seemed otherwise healthy. The pediatrician was hesitant to discourage the mother from breastfeeding by recommending she bottle-feed the baby; but clearly, something needed to be done to help the baby gain weight. The pediatrician wondered if I could recommend a breastfeeding-friendly solution. I was eager to speak with the mother, who told me her newborn had been sleeping for long periods during the day. When he eventually awoke, he was too agitated to effectively breastfeed. The reason for the baby's weight loss was obvious; this well-intentioned mother had not breastfed often enough over the last few days.

My advice to the mother was simple. To encourage frequent feeding, I suggested she hold her son close throughout the day. Holding her son calmed him, and he began actively breastfeeding. Happily, this strategy worked, and the baby regained the weight he had lost in just a few days. This story has a happy ending because the pediatrician sought a solution that strengthened her patient's breastfeeding relationship. Had this doctor not valued breastfeeding, she may have advised the mother to bottle-feed formula to her baby, which may have led the mother to abandon breastfeeding altogether.

BE AWARE OF MISINFORMATION THAT CAN HARM YOUR BREASTFEEDING EFFORTS

Unfortunately, not all medical professionals are aware of the significant benefits breastfeeding provides to the health of their clients. I once heard of an obstetrician's office holding monthly raffles to give away baskets of infant formula, bottles, and pacifiers. Please, if you encounter such a practice, run away as fast as safely possible! Another reason to be sure your obstetrician or midwife is a breastfeeding ally is that he or she will continue to provide your medical care for six weeks after you have your baby, which is a critical time in establishing your breastfeeding relationship. The wrong breastfeeding advice at this time can be devastating. This is exactly what happened to Paula and her baby, Brittany.

Paula called my home office with a sad story. On the advice of her obstetrician, she had not breastfed her two-week-old daughter, Brittany, for ten days. When Brittany was three days old, Paula became ill, and her obstetrician had prescribed the antibiotic clindamycin. The doctor told Paula the drug was incompatible with breastfeeding. Paula stopped breastfeeding Brittany and began giving her formula bottles. Paula went on to explain that she had occasionally pumped during this time, but to my dismay, she had thrown all of the milk away. Now that she had finished the antibiotic, her milk supply had dwindled, and Brittany had forgotten how to breastfeed.

Paula and Brittany's breastfeeding relationship was needlessly jeopardized by her doctor's incorrect information. The antibiotic clindamycin is safe for breastfeeding mothers, and Paula could have continued to breastfeed Brittany while taking the medication and recovering from the infection. Paula's unfortunate situation could have been avoided if her obstetrician had referred to Dr. Hale's *Medications and Mothers' Milk*. Had the doctor consulted this widely available reference book before counseling Paula, she would have seen that clindamycin is approved by the AAP for breastfeeding mothers because almost none of the drug passes into breast milk.[6]

If a mother needs a medication that poses a true risk to her breastfeeding baby, it is often possible to find an alternate medication that is safe for breastfeeding. However, as the following example illustrates, sometimes a medical situation necessitates a break in breastfeeding. I met Janice soon after the birth of her daughter, Ruth. During our visit, Janice shared her amazing story with me. Five years ago, she was diagnosed with a rare cancer. Janice had surgery and chemotherapy. Incredibly she recovered and is now a first-time mother. I was captivated by Janice's story as well as her sense of humor and easy smile.

Janice's follow-up care requires that she periodically undergo full body scans. These PET scans include the injection of a contrast dye. Some contrast agents are safe while breastfeeding; however, the substance Janice was scheduled to receive would require a break from breastfeeding. Janice was given conflicting information about how long after the scan she would need to wait before breastfeeding. Doctors, nurses, and radiologists all told her something different. I consulted the Drug Clearing House in Rochester, New York, a resource available to clinicians, and determined that Janice would need to wait twenty-four hours after her scan before breastfeeding Ruth. During that time, Janice pumped and discarded her breast milk. Meanwhile, Ruth took bottles of pumped breast milk that Janice had previously prepared. The good news is that Janice has remained cancer-free and continues to be a breastfeeding mother.

HOW DO I KNOW IF THE MEDICATION I AM TAKING IS SAFE?

The fact that a drug is available for over-the-counter (OTC) purchase is not an indicator of the drug's safety for breastfeeding mothers. The OTC decongestant commonly known as Sudafed (pseudoephedrine) can significantly decrease a mother's milk supply. Most of my clients would prefer a stuffy nose to a depressed milk supply!

The fact that a medication is available only by prescription does not necessarily mean that it is unsafe for a breastfeeding mother. There are many factors to consider when determining if a drug is appropriate for a breastfeeding mother. Most mothers are not aware that many medications given to adults are also given to babies in pediatric doses. As a general rule, if a medication can be given to a baby, then it is usually safe for a mother to take while breastfeeding.

The antifungal medication, Diflucan (fluconazole), is an example of a medication that is safe for breastfeeding mothers and babies.[7] Diflucan is useful for treating a painful condition called ductal candidiasis in breastfeeding mothers as well as thrush infections in babies. It is helpful to understand the particular properties of a drug and how the drug interacts with a mother's body. Drugs that are protein bound circulate in the mother's system and are unlikely to enter breast milk. Sometimes the molecular size and structure of a particular drug prohibits its passage into breast milk, as is the case with the anticoagulant drug heparin.[8] Finally, it is important to consider the age of the baby and the amount of breast milk the baby is receiving. Premature infants may be more sensitive to certain medications present in breast milk than healthy term babies.

As these examples show, it is important to seek up-to-date information in regard to medication and breastfeeding. When determining if a drug is appropriate for a breastfeeding mother, a breastfeeding ally refers to *Medications and Mothers' Milk*—not the *Physicians' Desk Reference (PDR)*. The right information can go a long way in preserving your breastfeeding relationship, whereas the wrong information can quickly harm it.

HOW CAN I RECOGNIZE A BREASTFEEDING ALLY?

Keep an open mind while you are looking for a breastfeeding ally. Instead of a traditional pediatrician some of my clients take their baby to a family practice doctor who knows the medical history of the entire family. Many practices use nurse practitioners and physician assistants (PAs) as members of the office team. In most states, nurse practitioners and PAs can assess, diagnose, and treat illnesses, and with the appropriate training can give supportive breastfeeding advice. Make arrangements to visit with any perspective pediatrician before your baby is born. Prenatal consultations are an opportunity to get acquainted with the office, the staff, and the doctor.

During the visit, look at the office, listen to how the doctor answers your questions, and notice how you feel.

Look at the pediatrician's office space

An office space displaying pictures of babies bottle-feeding or posters with formula company logos are red flags signaling a medical practice that views formula feeding as the norm. Furthermore, doctors who distribute formula samples and formula gift bags have bought into pharmaceutical advertising and cannot be trusted for current breastfeeding advice.

Listen to how the pediatrician answers the following questions

To avoid receiving unsupportive advice later, learn to ask the right questions now. Knowing what questions to ask when interviewing a pediatrician will reveal whether he or she is a breastfeeding ally. These questions are meant to guide your discussion and reflect the concerns my clients have shared with me over the years.

- *Will the doctor visit you and your baby at the hospital?* Find out if the doctor has hospital privileges where your baby will be born. Specifically ask if the doctor shares hospital responsibilities with anyone else in the office or with another group of doctors. Many parents have told me that they were disappointed when a doctor other than their chosen pediatrician showed up at the hospital the morning after their baby was born.
- *Will the doctor agree to examine your baby in your hospital room instead of the newborn nursery?* The newborn physical exam consists of a head-to-toe examination of your baby. The doctor will feel your baby's head and look at your baby's eyes, ears, mouth, skin, and muscle tone. In addition, the doctor will listen to your baby's heart, lungs, and belly sounds. Besides avoiding separation from your baby, having the exam conducted in your

room allows you the opportunity to get to know your baby and pediatrician better. As one of my clients remarked, "I loved seeing the pediatrician interact with my baby."

- *Will the pediatrician be recommending or ordering any routine supplements for your baby in the hospital?* Routine feedings of sugar water, sterile water, or formula are not recommended for breastfeeding babies. Furthermore, bottle nipples and pacifiers can interfere with your newborn's ability to breastfeed. If your baby is breastfeeding frequently, then supplements should not be necessary. Your colostrum is the perfect food for your new baby.

- *Will the doctor give you up-to-date breastfeeding advice?* A sure sign of a breastfeeding ally is a pediatrician who is a La Leche League medical associate, which means that he or she regularly receives resource materials appropriate to supporting breastfeeding in an office setting. These references enable office staff to give breastfeeding-friendly advice to new mothers. A pediatrician with many breastfed babies in his practice told me, "These reference books are a must in my office."

- *Will the doctor recommend you breastfeed whenever your baby signals hunger?* Babies don't wear watches because they can't tell time! However, your healthy baby will let you know when he or she feels hungry. It's normal for your baby to breastfeed at frequent intervals during the day and at night. Scheduled and timed feedings are based on a formula and bottle-feeding mentality rather than breastfeeding physiology. Doctors who recommend limiting your baby's time or frequency of feeding cannot be considered breastfeeding allies.

Notice how you feel after your visit

After visiting the office and meeting the doctor, notice how you feel. You should feel comfortable enough to share any future concerns about your baby's health with the doctor. If not, keep looking. Eventually you will find a breastfeeding ally.

BUILDING A COMMUNITY OF BREASTFEEDING ALLIES

Several years ago, my friend Evelyn got married and moved across the country. Within a year, Evelyn and her husband had a daughter named Beth. When I called to ask Evelyn how it felt to be a new mother, I was surprised when Evelyn told me she found motherhood "very lonely." Years later, when I married and had children of my own, I remembered Evelyn's words and found them to be true. As a new mother, my life revolved around holding my baby, breastfeeding, and changing my baby's diapers. Although I loved my new role, I sorely missed the camaraderie of my friends from work.

Whether you live in spread-out suburbia or a crowded city, you need not breastfeed your baby in isolation. Breastfeeding hormones, particularly oxytocin, are the same hormones that cause us to feel accepted and affiliated in social situations.[9] That means breastfeeding is meant to be socially shared! Cecelia was pregnant for the first time and eager for breastfeeding information, so I suggested she attend a La Leche League meeting before her baby's birth. During her first meeting, Cecelia enjoyed watching the other mothers breastfeed their babies as the leader answered questions from the group. The following month Cecelia returned to the meeting with her brand-new baby, Maddie. Cecelia later told me, "Everyone rallied around me and Maddie. It felt great to have so much support."

In addition to breastfeeding support groups, you can forge connections with other mothers in a variety of ways. When leaving a yoga class one morning, I happened to pass the gymnasium where an aerobics instructor was leading a group of new moms through some exercises. Meanwhile, some of the babies slept in their strollers while other babies played on a large blanket spread out on the gym floor. As I watched the class, the moms took breaks to care for their babies and then rejoined the class. Later, I ran into these same moms and babies enjoying each other's company at Starbucks. Several of these women had been clients of mine, and I was happy to see them surrounded by social support.

Special situations call for specialized support. Mother-to-mother support is especially valuable to mothers of twins or triplets. When working with a mother who is breastfeeding twins, I do my best to convince her to contact a support group geared toward parenting twins. I also put her in contact with another client of mine who has successfully breastfed her twins. A breastfeeding mother of twins needs the heartfelt inspiration only another mother of twins can provide.

SUMMARY OF BREASTFEEDING ABCs

As you prepare to become a breastfeeding mother, plan to surround yourself with breastfeeding allies. It is important to have an obstetrician who is knowledgeable about breastfeeding because he or she will continue to provide your medical care after your baby is born. Don't make the mistake of choosing a pediatrician for reasons of convenience alone. Take time to look at the office and ask the right questions. Breastfeeding allies are everywhere; make breastfeeding a social experience by reaching out to other mothers.

A. ALLIES

Find health-care providers who are breastfeeding allies. During prenatal visits, your obstetrician or midwife should discuss the benefits that breastfeeding provides to your health. When determining if a medication is safe for a breastfeeding mother, a breastfeeding ally consults *Medications and Mothers' Milk* not the *PDR*. A pediatrician should be able to provide you with accurate up-to-date breastfeeding advice and refer complicated breastfeeding problems that he or she cannot answer to a lactation consultant.

B. BUILD

Build a community of breastfeeding support. Wherever you live, chances are you can attend a breastfeeding support group where you will meet other new mothers. Attending a meeting before your baby is born will give you the chance to see mothers breastfeeding their babies and strengthen your positive breastfeeding mindset.

C. CONNECT

After your baby is born, seek social support; there is no reason for you to breastfeed in isolation. Stay connected to other mothers. Look for ways to meet new mothers with your baby. Join a mother-and-baby exercise class or a playgroup. Chances are many of the mothers are breastfeeding their babies and will support your breastfeeding efforts. Breastfeeding hormones are the same hormones that lead us to socialize and affiliate with one another. Sharing your experiences with other mothers can add to your enjoyment of breastfeeding.

CHAPTER THREE

Planning for a Gentle Birth

"I had no idea that giving birth would
become so complicated."

—Ann

always begin a consultation by asking a new client to describe her baby's birth. Most new mothers are surprised by my question and are completely unaware of how labor and birth can affect their breastfeeding experience. Ann's birth story is an example of how a negative birth experience can end a breastfeeding experience before it even begins.

I met Ann five days after her first child, Jarod, was born by an unplanned cesarean section. Ann and her husband were new to the area when she became pregnant. Ann sailed easily through her pregnancy without so much as a day of nausea. The couple did little to prepare for labor and birth. Ann assumed her baby would be born naturally and that she would breastfeed her baby just as her sister and friends had.

Ann's pale blue eyes filled with tears as she told me what happened when she arrived at the hospital in active labor. "I didn't know what was wrong, but the doctor said that I did not labor fast enough, and they ordered that I have an IV drip, and then the doctor broke my baby's water sack with a long needle." Ann sobbed as she described how helpless she felt being wheeled toward the operating room for an emergency cesarean

29

section. "It was all wrong. I was all wrong, and I knew that it was the wrong way for my baby to be born. When I finally saw my baby, he had a pacifier in his mouth, and I was in so much pain that I couldn't hold him even though I wanted to more than anything else in the world." Despite my best efforts, Ann was never able to successfully breastfeed Jarod. My home visits, follow-up phone calls, and written breastfeeding plans could not compete with the demoralizing memory of her son's disappointing birth.

Perhaps things would have turned out differently if Ann had not gotten caught up in the cascade of medical interventions so common in modern obstetrics. Although natural birth and breastfeeding were critically important to Ann, she was both uninformed and unprepared to make her vision a reality. Not knowing what else to do, she passively consented to a series of interventions that ultimately robbed her of the birth that she imagined.

Gentle birth means having your baby with as few routine medical interventions as possible. Although labor can be an unpredictable adventure, you can take steps that lead to a gentle birth. In today's high-tech society, few parents realize that they have choices about labor and birth, and that these choices have a tremendous impact on the breastfeeding experience.

WILL ROUTINE LABOR MEDICATIONS AFFECT MY BABY?

Labor is an experience you and your almost born baby share. The two of you are a team. Your labor contractions help your baby shift into perfect position for birth, and the labor process prepares your baby's lungs for that first breath of earthly air. It is important to remember that during labor you and your baby are linked by your placenta. Naturally, any medication you take while in labor, including epidural pain medication, will travel through the placenta and reach your baby.[1] Because of variances in body weight, metabolism, and medication dosing, it is difficult to predict exactly how labor medications will affect your baby. This is why the same dose of the narcotic pain reliever Stadol, administered to one mother during active labor causes her baby to be sleepy upon birth, while the same medication given to the mother in an adjoining labor room has no noticeable effect on her newborn.

CAN I HAVE AN EPIDURAL *AND* A GENTLE BIRTH?

Eva, a first-time mother, was nervous about what the labor process would entail. As her labor slowly progressed, she felt herself becoming tense and claustrophobic. When one contraction finished, Eva found herself unable to rest, fearing the inevitable sensation that the next contraction would bring. Eva became helplessly caught up in an escalating cycle of fear, tension, and pain. Nothing her husband or the labor and delivery nurse did seemed to help. Finally, the anesthesiologist gave Eva an epidural. Shortly after receiving the epidural, the fear receded, and Eva was able to enjoy giving birth to Emma. Looking back, Eva describes her epidural as "the right decision at the right time."

Like Eva, many of my clients have told me that epidural pain relief helped them to relax and progress through the next stage of their labor. Gentle birth does not necessarily mean a natural birth without any medications or interventions. At the same time, an epidural is not without risk, and having one may or may not help you in your quest for a gentle birth. Epidurals contain a combination of medications given by continuous infusion into the epidural space of a mother's lower back. An epidural contains both an anesthetic such as Bupivacaine and a narcotic such as Fentanyl.[2] These drugs work together to rapidly relieve labor pain.

However, as my client Sheri describes, epidurals are not without consequences. Sheri had not made any specific plans for her birth and was not aware of how an epidural would affect her labor. "I had been in labor for a few hours before going to the hospital. After my doctor examined me, she said that I had a long way to go before Brenden would be born, and she suggested that I have an epidural. Since I was beginning to get uncomfortable and didn't know what else to do, I agreed to have the epidural."

Along with pain relief, epidurals cause a mother to lose sensation in her legs, forcing her to labor in bed. The numbness also inhibits a mother's ability to urinate, necessitating the insertion of a urinary catheter during labor. Sheri continued, "The pain was gone, but my legs were numb, and the nurse had to catheterize me two times because my bladder got so full." Having an epidural tends to slow down the entire labor process.[3] This often leads to an intervention such as the artificial rupture of membranes or the administration of the drug Pitocin to reinvigorate labor contractions. Sheri described what happened next. "After a few hours, the nurse checked me and since I had not made much progress, the doctor ordered Pitocin to move things along. It seemed to work, and soon the nurses told me I could start pushing. This was difficult because I couldn't feel when and where to push. Eventually, the doctor used a vacuum cup on top of Brenden's head to pull him out."

Sometimes, as Sheri experienced, an epidural dampens a mother's ability to work with her contractions during the pushing stage of labor, leading to vacuum extraction of her baby or ultimately a cesarean section. Of additional concern, epidurals frequently cause a mother and her baby to have a fever.[4] Since fever can be a sign of illness, this may lead to a mother being unexpectedly separated from her newborn while medical staff investigate the cause of the fever.

DO LABOR MEDICATIONS AFFECT BREASTFEEDING?

It is difficult to quantify how labor medications affect a newborn's ability to breastfeed. However, studies have shown that babies born following an unmedicated birth are more alert and begin effectively breastfeeding sooner than babies born after exposure to labor medications.[5] Babies born to mothers who had multiple birth interventions such as IV narcotics, epidurals, and vacuum extractions had the most difficulty beginning to breastfeed.[6] This lack of effective breastfeeding during the immediate new-born period can lead a baby to lose excessive weight.[7] It is important for mothers to know that receiving multiple medications, interventions, or a cesarean section may cause a delay in their body's ability to produce mature breast milk.[8]

WHAT IS GENTLE BIRTH?

My definition of gentle birth is two-fold. Besides giving birth with as few interventions as possible, a gentle birth involves identifying an aspect of your baby's upcoming birth that is very important to you. Perhaps you want the sensation of touching the top of your baby's head the moment before birth, or you may want to be the one who cuts the umbilical cord that has joined the two of you together. Connecting with an important event during your baby's birth allows you the opportunity to create a positive birth experience. Once you are aware of what is important, you can begin to devise a plan to realize your goal.

Monica is an example of a mother who used the concept of gentle birth to fulfill a particular dream that went unrealized during a cesarean birth of her first child. Pregnant with her second child, Monica wanted this baby to be placed directly on her abdomen upon birth. This would be impossible if Monica had another cesarean section. If Monica was going to hold her just born baby belly to belly, then she would need to give birth vaginally. With the help of an experienced doula (a professional labor assistant), Monica devised a birth plan to overcome the circumstances that led to her previous cesarean section. As with her first daughter, Monica's labor was long and tiring, but at last Grace was born and, as planned, placed directly on her mother's warm skin.

Sometimes it is something so seemingly small that makes a birth memorable. On a personal note, when my second baby was born, I wanted to be the one to announce his gender. I don't know why but this was very important to me. Honoring my request, at the moment of birth, everyone in the room fell silent and waited for me to pick up my baby and state, "It's a boy!" I cried then and five years later, the memory of that amazing moment brings back joyful tears. Had I not connected with my wish and made it known, any member of my well-intentioned birth team might have called out Max's gender, and my dream would have gone unrealized.

HOW DO I PLAN A GENTLE BIRTH?

There are four steps you can use to guide you in planning your gentle birth.

Connect with your "golden moment"

Close your eyes and imagine your baby's upcoming birth. As the birth unfolds in your mind, notice what moment is most important to you. Think about what special memory you want to create for you and your baby. What role do you see yourself playing in creating this special memory? As you imagine your baby's birth, it may help to read *Ina May's Guide to Childbirth* by Ina May Gaskin. These powerful birth stories will offer you a fresh perspective on childbirth. The unique exercises in Pam England and Rob Horowitz's book, *Birthing from Within,* are designed to prepare you for the emotional and physical aspects of birth and may help you discover the golden moment in your baby's birth. Whether it's wearing your own nightgown in the hospital or playing certain music as your baby is born, once you realize what is important to you, write it down. You will use what you have discovered to plan your baby's gentle birth.

Choose a childbirth educator

Gentle birth requires preparation. Before automatically registering for the childbirth class offered through the hospital, consider a class taught by an independent childbirth educator. Because an independent childbirth educator is not employed by the hospital, she is more apt to give unbiased information about medical interventions. She will help you learn to birth with fewer medications and teach you and your partner techniques to help your labor progress naturally. When searching for a childbirth class, investigate all the options available in your area. Finding the right instructor will go a long way in helping you to realize your goal of a gentle birth.

Instructors certified in the Bradley Method® of natural childbirth teach husbands and partners how to effectively coach a mother through an unmedicated labor and birth. The Bradley Method® emphasizes good prenatal nutrition, relaxation during labor, and self-advocacy in the hospital. The Association of Labor Assistants and Childbirth Educators (ALACE) certifies labor doulas and childbirth educators. Rather than following a specific method, ALACE instructors have an eclectic approach and teach a wide variety of techniques to cope with the intensity of labor. Hypno-Birthing teaches a mother to profoundly relax during childbirth by practicing self-hypnosis. By achieving a deep state of relaxation, a mother is able to minimize the pain and fear associated with birth.

Consider a doula

A doula is professional labor assistant. Doulas are trained to physically and emotionally support a mother and her partner through the ups and downs of labor and birth. To an experienced doula, supporting gentle birth is as natural as breathing. During labor, she may recommend therapeutic position changes, massage, or aromatherapy. Most important of all, a doula offers constant companionship. First-time parents Kristin and Keith described their doula as "still by our side when the nurses changed shift, constantly reassuring us that our labor was going really well." The research is clear; mothers who have a doula join the birth team have shorter labors, need less medication, and have fewer cesarean sections.[9]

Compose a birth plan

A birth plan is a roadmap summarizing the steps leading to your goal of gentle birth. Your birth plan should clearly describe the golden moment you want to capture during your baby's birth. Keep the plan short; hospital personnel are naturally caring people but they are very busy and will not have time to sift through a birth plan that is longer than one page. Remember, the document does not control the process of birth; rather it will help you and your birth team work together. For example, in Josephine's birth plan, she requested that the lights be dimmed during birth in the hope that baby Jesse would open his eyes as he was being born. Happy to make this happen, Josephine's nurse turned down the bright spotlight over the hospital bed. When writing your birth plan, look for input from your childbirth educator and doula. Consult www.birthplan.com to learn more about writing a birth plan. If your doctor or midwife is a breastfeeding ally, he or she will be open to reviewing your completed birth plan.

CAN A CESAREAN SECTION BE A GENTLE BIRTH?

When I met Nell for a prenatal consultation, she was just two weeks shy of her due date. Pregnant for the first time, Nell looked healthy and full of life. However, her smile quickly faded, and her glowing face darkened when she told me that her doctors were planning to deliver her baby by cesarean section, "That's not the way my husband and I had planned to bring our baby into the world."

Instead of turning into a head-down position, Nell's unborn baby was in a breech position. About 4 percent of babies don't assume a vertex or head-down position and will approach birth with either their bottom or feet toward the birth canal.[10] In recent years, obstetricians have made a habit of delivering breech babies by cesarean section either because they don't have the experience or because they don't want to assume the risk of supporting the mother through natural birth.[11] Nell's doctor had tried to help her baby turn but the version technique did not work, and her baby remained in breech position.

As the days passed, Nell resigned herself to having a cesarean section and decided against alternative therapies such as acupuncture or chiropractic maneuvers to change her baby's position. Meanwhile, we devised a plan to make Nell's cesarean section as gentle a birth as possible. The day before her scheduled cesarean section, Nell went into labor at home. On the way to the hospital, Nell was excited to feel her body working, and these early labor contractions helped prepare her baby for birth. As planned, Nell had spinal anesthesia and was awake during the surgery. Nell had a healthy eight-pound girl named Justina, and as Nell requested in her birth plan, Justina was brought to her within minutes of birth so Nell could see and touch her baby. With the support of her nurses and her husband, Nell held Justina in the recovery room and began breastfeeding even before she was transferred to the hospital's postpartum unit. Although Nell was disappointed with having a cesarean section, the plans she made to ease Justina's entry into the world by greeting her as soon as possible and welcoming her with close holding paid off. By preparing to make her cesarean section as gentle as possible, Nell and Justina went on to develop a close breastfeeding relationship.

WILL HAVING A GENTLE BIRTH PREVENT ALL BREASTFEEDING PROBLEMS?

I had briefly spoken by phone with Kimberly while she was pregnant and developing her birth plan. Kimberly and her husband, Doug, had hired a doula to support them in labor and were excited about becoming parents for the first time. Several weeks later, the couple called to report that Gabrielle was born following a rapid labor and natural birth. Now that she was home from the hospital, Kimberly was having a difficult time breastfeeding Gabrielle.

The next day I went to visit the family and found that Kimberly had significant bruising and bleeding on both nipples. During the consultation, I assisted Kimberly with positioning Gabrielle for feeding, and I prescribed ointments for Kimberly's nipples. Over the next few days, Kimberly healed and Gabrielle became a better breastfeeder. Because Kimberly had a gentle birth, she had the energy to focus on quickly solving her breastfeeding difficulty. Likewise, Gabrielle remained alert and was able to learn to breastfeed without causing her mother further nipple trauma. Gentle birth may not prevent all breastfeeding problems, but if problems arise, you will be fortified by your positive birth experience to work toward a solution.

Although not impossible, it is more challenging to cope with a breast-feeding problem while simultaneously recovering from a difficult birth. When Becky went past her due date without going into labor, she was admitted to the hospital to be induced. Two days after starting the induction process, her labor rapidly progressed, but once fully dilated, Becky encountered difficulty and ended up having an emergency cesarean section. Becky finally arrived home with baby Emily after spending nearly a week in the hospital.

During our consultation, I could tell Becky had been through an ordeal. She was pale and exhausted. Becky's feet and ankles were so swollen that her slippers did not fit, and she had painful purple bruises on both arms where her IV had been. Becky was discouraged because she was not making much milk, and baby Emily was still losing weight. I explained to Becky that her milk production was suppressed due to her long arduous labor and cesarean birth. Determined to work through this difficulty, Becky began regularly using an electric breast pump to stimulate her milk supply. While Becky worked on increasing her milk supply, we devised a plan to supplement Emily with her mother's pumped breast milk.

Unfortunately, several days later, Becky developed an infection along her incision site that required antibiotics and daily dressing changes. As she recovered from this unexpected setback, Becky never lost sight of her breastfeeding goal. Her progress was slow, but Becky healed from her birth, built up her milk supply, and is still breastfeeding Emily.

SUMMARY OF BREASTFEEDING ABCs

As you can see, your baby's birth experience will have an effect on your future breastfeeding relationship. Take time during your pregnancy to plan for a gentle birth. Create a positive birth experience by discovering an aspect of your birth that is most important to you, and devise a plan to realize that goal. No method is foolproof, but with less medication and fewer interventions to recover from, you and your baby will have more energy to focus on breastfeeding.

A. AWARENESS

Develop an awareness of what is most important to you about your baby's birth. As you imagine your baby's upcoming birth, notice what aspect of the birth you most want to experience. This is your golden moment during your baby's birth. It may be wearing your own clothes instead of a hospital gown or being the first one to say your baby's name. Once you uncover your golden moment, write it down and plan your birth so that you can realize your vision. Realizing this goal will give you a feeling of accomplishment and create a positive memory of your baby's birth.

B. BIRTH OPTIONS

Give birth with as few medications and interventions as possible. Gentle birth will make breastfeeding easier for you and your baby. Gentle birth requires some preparation, so look for a childbirth educator to teach you a variety of techniques that support gentle birth. Consider hiring a doula as part of your birth team. Mothers who have the support of a trained doula have fewer medications and interventions during birth.

C. COMPOSE

Compose a birth plan. A birth plan is a concise one-page document outlining the steps you and your partner plan to take during labor and birth. Your birth plan should clearly describe the golden moment that you want to realize during birth. By design, your birth plan will help your doctors and nurses understand how they can assist you in having a positive birth experience. As you compose your birth plan, ask for input from your childbirth educator and doula. If you have a cesarean section, plan to see and touch your baby as soon as possible.

CHAPTER FOUR

How to Hold Your Baby After Birth

"After my baby was born,
I didn't know what to do next."
—IRENE

rene's labor was quickly drawing to a close. It was nearly noon, and she had been experiencing contractions since the previous evening. As specified in her birth plan, Irene wanted to try a variety of comfort measures during active labor before having an epidural. With the support of her husband, Charles, Irene walked, sat on the birth ball, and took a shower to cope with her labor contractions. Finally the couple was about to get a glimpse of their first baby. With Irene's next effort, they could see their baby's thick black hair, then a face emerged, followed by a shoulder, and all at once their baby was born! The wet baby let out a loud wail as the obstetrician lifted him onto a towel draped over Irene's abdomen. Just before the nurse scooped up the towel containing the baby, Irene and Charles could see that their baby was a boy whom they would call Joshua.

The nurse deposited the bundle under the radiant warmer in the corner of the room and began rubbing the baby dry. Next, she set about the task of weighing, measuring, and monitoring Joshua as he lay beneath the hospital heat lamps. Meanwhile, the obstetrician finished up with Irene and left the room in a hurry for the next delivery. From her hospital bed,

Irene strained to see her baby. Still beneath the warmer, Joshua was now dressed in a diaper and a hospital-issue white T-shirt, and a blue hat covered his black hair. Although his eyes were open, Joshua's vision was temporarily blurred by an antibiotic ointment routinely administered to all newborns. The nurse assured Irene and Charles that Joshua was a healthy baby weighing in at seven pounds two ounces and measuring nineteen inches long. Charles began taking pictures of Joshua under the warmer, and Irene began making phone calls to share the good news. A while later, the nurse presented Irene with her baby expertly swaddled and sound asleep. Looking at Joshua asleep in his bundle of blankets, Irene wondered when she should start breastfeeding.

This scenario repeats itself over and over again in both rushed inner-city hospitals and rural community health-care centers across the country. Without realizing it, mothers and babies are missing out on the first step leading to future breastfeeding harmony: prolonged skin-to-skin holding after birth. Given enough time, newborns have been shown to crawl toward their mother's breast and begin nursing without assistance.[1] For a mother, this skin-to-skin experience releases hormones associated with the production of milk and feelings of attachment toward her new baby.[2] By learning how to hold your baby, you will be empowered to begin your breastfeeding relationship within the first crucial hours after birth.

Skin-to-skin holding is the bridge between your baby's birth and the beginning of your future breastfeeding relationship. The aforementioned couple, Irene and Charles, took the necessary steps to prepare for Joshua's gentle birth. They chose a childbirth class that taught them a variety of coping techniques, which they successfully employed during Irene's labor. As planned, Irene had an epidural later in labor, lessening the time that she and her baby were exposed to medication. However, once Joshua was born, they had not made plans to welcome him with skin-to-skin holding. Irene intended to breastfeed Joshua but instead of laying the groundwork for future breastfeeding success, she lost precious hours after birth to hospital procedures and protocol. When Irene finally held Joshua, he had been lulled into a very deep sleep by the artificial heat of the hospital warmer and a tight blanket swaddle. Because the nurse gave Joshua his eye ointment before he had the opportunity to spend time with his parents, Irene, Charles, and Joshua missed gazing into each other's eyes after birth.

WHAT IS SKIN-TO-SKIN HOLDING?

Skin-to-skin contact means holding your naked or diaper-clad newborn against your naked chest. As shown in Illustration 1, when in a skin-to-skin embrace, your baby's belly should be snuggled between your breasts. Your baby's head should be turned to one side and above the level of your

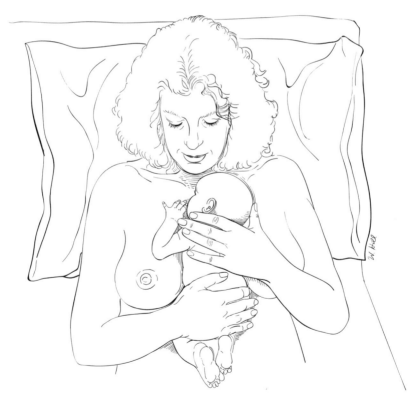

Illustration 1. Skin-to-skin holding

breasts and resting comfortably beneath your chin. A blanket can cover you as a couple.

IS SKIN-TO-SKIN HOLDING BETTER THAN
THE HOSPITAL WARMER?

One of the responsibilities of a neonatal nurse practitioner in the neonatal intensive care unit (NICU) is to rapidly respond to the delivery room beeper. Sometimes an obstetrician or a labor and delivery nurse will request the nurse practitioner on-call to evaluate a baby after it is born. I remember being called to see a baby boy who was about one hour old and beginning to show signs of respiratory distress. Although it was dark upon entering the delivery suite, I could see both parents wore worried expressions on their faces. They had been told their baby, Ethan, might need to be admitted to the NICU to evaluate his abnormal breathing.

Baby Ethan lay flat on his back under the hospital's radiant warmer. With his eyes tightly shut and his forehead wrinkled, Ethan looked more like a little old man than a newborn baby. Above his head, the heating element in the warmer glowed red hot while the examination light cast a sterile white aura over his body. The entire unit let out a shrill alarm as it repeatedly failed to register Ethan's temperature from a probe that had become detached from his skin.

As I looked Ethan over and listened to his chest with a stethoscope, I was reassured by his normal heart sounds and by the fact that he was moving air well. Although he was breathing rapidly and making a distressing grunting sound, Ethan's color was pink, and he was not in need of oxygen. Neither Ethan's birth record nor his mother's medical history contained anything out of the ordinary. I concluded that Ethan was having a difficult time adjusting to life outside the security of his mother's womb. Naturally, the best person to guide him through this time of transition was his own mother. I explained my findings to Ethan's parents and assured his mother that she was the best medicine for her son. Next, I prescribed skin-to-skin holding and placed Ethan under his mother's hospital gown. The labor and delivery nurse agreed to help keep Ethan continually against his mother's skin for the next hour.

Once in skin-to-skin contact with his mother, Ethan immediately opened his eyes. Twenty minutes later, his rapid breathing slowed and his distressing grunts became less frequent. When I checked in on the family an hour later, Ethan's symptoms of distress were gone and replaced by signs of feeding readiness. Ethan's parents were thrilled that their new baby would not need to spend the night in the NICU.

Dr. Nils Bergman has proven that skin-to-skin holding is powerful life-saving medicine.[3] Dr. Bergman dramatically improved the outcome of premature babies in Africa by keeping them in constant contact with their mothers. Babies receiving his method of Kangaroo Mother Care were better able to digest their mother's breast milk, achieve healthy sleep patterns, and leave the hospital sooner than babies cared for in incubators. If your baby needs special medical care, ask the medical team when it will be safe for you to hold your baby skin-to-skin. It is often possible to hold your baby while he or she is receiving IV fluid or oxygen.

WILL SKIN-TO-SKIN HOLDING HELP ME BREASTFEED?

Given enough uninterrupted time in the skin-to-skin position, healthy newborns will move toward their mother's breast and begin breastfeeding without assistance. For this reason, the American Academy of Pediatrics recommends that labor and delivery units postpone routine hospital procedures like infant weighing and washing until after a mother and her baby have had undisturbed time together.[4] These procedures can be done later when they won't interrupt a newborn's natural progression along the skin-to-skin continuum leading to breastfeeding.

Being physically close to your baby stimulates your body to release the hormone oxytocin, which primes the flow of your colostrum, and later on initiates the flow of your mature milk. Once your breastfeeding relationship is established, oxytocin is responsible for causing your milk to leak whenever you think about your baby or hear your baby cry. This is why I begin the hands-on phase of every client consultation by placing a mother and baby together in the skin-to-skin position. Leaking some breast milk while in this position reassures a client who is having breast-feeding difficulty that her body is ready to breastfeed even before her baby is positioned at the breast.

Once in skin-to-skin position, most healthy hungry babies will begin turning their head from side to side, as they launch themselves toward their mother's breast. These are signals that your baby is ready to breastfeed. Your baby is literally searching for your breast. After a full feeding, returning your baby to the skin-to-skin position helps your baby to digest your breast milk and achieve a healthy sleep state. In fact, I often end a consultation in the same way in which it began, with a mother and her baby in a skin-to-skin embrace. Sometimes I do little else during a consultation but reinforce a client's already excellent mothering intuition.

This was the case when I met with Ellen and her baby, Ashley. Ashley was now twelve days old and Ellen's first baby. Ellen reported that since birth, Ashley had been inconsistent at the breast. Ashley would become agitated before feeding and have a difficult time getting attached. I asked Ellen to undress Ashley down to her diaper, and we weighed her on my scale. This process upset Ashley, and she began to cry. Next, I positioned Ashley in the skin-to-skin position with Ellen. I was happy to see Ellen instinctively place both hands firmly on her daughter's back. Comforted by her mother's touch, Ashley stopped crying. Ellen's body was also responding to the skin-to-skin position by leaking a good deal of breast milk. With Ashley now quiet and alert, I helped Ellen guide the baby toward her breast. In this composed state, Ashley attached well and breastfed vigorously. When the feeding was complete, Ellen instinctively lifted Ashley into the skin-to-skin position. Both mother and daughter responded so beautifully to skin-to-skin holding that I recommended Ellen begin and end as many feedings as possible with skin-to-skin holding.

Many newborns like Ashley are unable to breastfeed when they become upset by the sensation of their own hunger. The skin-to-skin position enabled Ashley to settle and calm herself enough to focus on learning to breastfeed. For Ashley, skin-to-skin holding eliminated the confusion she had previously associated with breastfeeding.

HOW DO I WELCOME MY BABY WITH SKIN-TO-SKIN HOLDING?

As mentioned previously, skin-to-skin contact means holding your newborn either naked or in a diaper on your naked chest between your breasts. Once positioned, a sheet or blanket can cover both of you. Skin-to-skin holding is the next step after birth leading to your breastfeeding relationship. As you and your baby get comfortable, the hormone oxytocin will automatically circulate in your body, naturally preparing you for the breastfeeding experience. The rhythm of your heart, the flow of your breath, and the scent of your skin all help to regulate your baby's biorhythms. The following steps will help guide you as you plan to welcome your baby after birth with skin-to-skin holding.

Touch your newborn

Make sure to add skin-to-skin holding after birth to your written birth plan. Most doctors and nurses will be eager to help you gently welcome your baby into the world if they know your plans.

Touching your baby is a continuation of gentle birth. When your baby is born, you and your husband or partner can help dry the wetness from your newborn's skin and hair. Drying your baby after birth helps to prevent your baby from becoming chilled. Next, ease your newborn into the skin-to-skin position. Be sure to remove your bra before snuggling your baby between your breasts and under your shirt or hospital gown. Your baby will naturally turn his or her head to one side. Once in position, your baby's head should end up beneath your chin. Continue to gently greet your newborn by firmly placing your hands on your baby's back. Welcome your baby into the world with skin-to-skin holding for as long as possible.

Your body heat will warm and comfort your baby. Hospital staff can easily check your baby's temperature and other vital signs while you hold your baby in this position. Dimming the lights in the hospital room will encourage your baby to open his or her eyes. Delaying the administration of routine eye ointment will make it possible for your baby to clearly see your face.

Talk to your newborn

While in the skin-to-skin position, welcome your newborn with your voice. Your baby will recognize the familiar sound of your voice. As you greet your baby, keep the lights in the hospital room low, so your baby can open his or her eyes and see your face. When I meet and hold a newborn during a consultation, I am repeatedly amazed to see the baby naturally gravitate toward the voices of his or her mother and father. Touching and talking to your new baby will naturally prepare your baby to breastfeed for the first time.

If your baby seems to move from the skin-to-skin position toward your breast, then you can help guide your baby toward the breast your baby has selected. Your newborn may not need any help with this first feeding. If your baby needs some help getting started, then bring your baby slightly below your breast with your nipple at the level of your baby's upper lip. This should signal your baby to open up and over your nipple. As your baby attaches to you, move your baby close to your body. Make sure you are comfortable; support your arm and wrist with a pillow.

Continue touching and talking to your newborn

Hold your baby in a skin-to-skin embrace as often as possible in the hours and days after birth. If you and your baby become separated by medical need or a hospital procedure, reestablish your connection through skin-to-skin holding. Being close to you and hearing your voice will help arouse an overly sleepy baby and also calm a frantic baby. Remember, the skin-to-skin position is the link between birth and breastfeeding.

WHAT IF I CAN'T HOLD MY NEWBORN AFTER BIRTH?

There are situations that will cause a delay in skin-to-skin holding after birth. If you are unable to hold your newborn because you are having a cesarean section or require medical attention, plan for an alternate holder. One of my clients, Julie, knew her second daughter, Leah, was going to be born by cesarean section. After Leah was born, Julie's husband, Kevin, welcomed his daughter into the world by holding her under his shirt. Leah was warm and perfectly content with her father and spent minimal time beneath the hospital warmer. Once Julie was settled in the recovery room, she was able to touch, hold, and breastfeed Leah.

The presence of meconium in your amniotic fluid will alter the sequence of events in the minutes after birth. Meconium is your newborn's first bowel movement. Sometimes a baby passes the green- or black-colored stool during the labor process. Although the presence of meconium does not usually indicate a problem, it is necessary for your baby to be properly suctioned. This procedure is best done before your baby has taken a breath, and it necessitates placing your newborn under the warmer. The process of suctioning your baby will take several minutes. Afterward, your baby should be returned to you for skin-to-skin holding.

USING SKIN-TO-SKIN HOLDING TO CALM YOUR CRYING NEWBORN

While working a weekend shift as a neonatal nurse practitioner, I went to visit a mother on the maternity floor to discuss her baby's lab tests. Both parents were relieved to hear that the lab results were normal. As we spoke, their baby, who was named Nolan, returned from the newborn nursery where he had undergone a repeat blood draw. As the patient care assistant wheeled the bassinet into the room, it was evident that Nolan was upset. With flailing arms and fisted hands, he had freed himself from his blanket swaddle. His eyes were tightly shut and his mouth was wide open in a tearless wail.

With their son back in the hospital room, the conversation turned to breastfeeding. Nolan's parents described their newborn as fussy, frequently out-of-sorts, and difficult to breastfeed. In fact, he had missed several feedings because he had been in and out of the newborn nursery having blood drawn. As we spoke, Nolan's cry reached a hysterical pitch, and his mother attempted to offer him a feeding at her breast. Nolan's parents agreed to let me help, and while his mother loosened her nightgown and removed her nursing bra, I undressed Nolan. Next, I showed Nolan's mother how to position him in a skin-to-skin hold.

Almost immediately, this seemed to be what Nolan needed. As Nolan quietly settled near his mother's heart, he returned her hug by extending both of his tiny arms across her chest. Soon Nolan and his mother were back in sync and able to breastfeed. Through frequent skin-to-skin holding, Nolan's parents discovered that their son was neither fussy nor difficult to manage; rather, Nolan was the calm and loving baby for whom they had wished.

USING SKIN-TO-SKIN HOLDING TO AROUSE YOUR SLEEPY NEWBORN

Sometimes a newborn is unable to breastfeed not because he or she is crying like Nolan, but because the baby has fallen into a very deep sleep. Although the situation seems to be at the opposite end of the spectrum from Nolan's example, the solution is mostly the same. This is the situation that new parents Irene and Charles found themselves in with baby Joshua. As described in the beginning of the chapter, Irene and Charles enjoyed the gentle birth of their son, Joshua. Although Irene and Joshua were healthy after birth, baby Joshua spent a great deal of time apart from Irene beneath the hospital warmer. When Irene finally held him, he was dressed, bundled in several blankets, and his vision was blurred by eye ointment. Under these conditions, there was little else Joshua could do but fall into a deep sleep. Because of the long delay in skin-to-skin contact, Irene and Joshua missed their initial opportunity to begin breastfeeding.

The good news is that it was not too late for a mother like Irene and a sleepy baby like Joshua to initiate a healthy breastfeeding relationship. The key was to awaken Joshua gently by releasing his tight swaddle and reuniting him with his mother in a skin-to-skin hold. The feel of Irene's heartbeat and breathing and the scent of his mother's skin reminded Joshua that he was hungry. Swaddling is a useful technique for calming a baby. However, in the initial hours and days following birth, a tight swaddle can induce such a deep sleep that newborns may miss the opportunity to breastfeed. Sometimes babies become sleepy following a long and difficult birth or a medical procedure. Skin-to-skin holding can help a baby overcome these hurdles and establish a breastfeeding relationship.

Skin-to-skin holding is the only technique that I employ to awaken a sleeping baby. Attempting to awaken your baby by pinching, tickling, or using a wet washcloth will cause your baby pain and teach your baby to recoil from your touch. It troubles me deeply that medical professionals still teach parents to awaken their baby for a feeding in this way because these annoyance techniques will damage your breastfeeding relationship by causing your baby to retreat from the breast. Remember, your breastfeeding relationship is built on a foundation of mutual love and trust. The best way to begin is by bringing your baby close to your heart in a skin-to-skin embrace.

SUMMARY OF BREASTFEEDING ABCs

By now, you know how powerful your touch is to your newborn. Your loving embrace is the link between your baby's birth and breastfeeding. Above all else, take your time as you greet your new baby. There is no reason to rush; you and your baby have waited a long time to meet at this moment. With your gentle guidance, your baby will acclimate to life outside the security of your womb. The rest of the world will wait.

A. ALIGN

Align your baby in the skin-to-skin position after birth. Touch your baby as soon as possible after birth by gently drying his or her skin. Lift your newborn's body into the skin-to-skin position. To benefit from the skin-to-skin experience, your baby should be naked or in a diaper, and you should remove your bra. Once properly aligned, your baby's body will be snuggled between your breasts. Your baby's head will turn to one side and will rest below your chin. Next, firmly place your hands on your baby's back. Once you are settled, a blanket can cover both of you.

B. BODY HEAT

Plan to let the natural heat of your body keep your newborn warm and comfortable. Following birth, your body heat is preferable to the artificial heat of the hospital's radiant warmer. Keep your baby close to you after birth instead of under the hospital warmer or wrapped up in a tight blanket swaddle. Your labor and delivery nurse can easily monitor your baby's temperature and other vital signs while you hold your baby in the skin-to-skin position. If your baby needs special care, it may still be possible to hold your baby while he or she receives IV fluids or oxygen.

C. CONTINUE

Continue holding your newborn in skin-to-skin contact for as long as possible. Postpone nonemergency routine hospital procedures like weighing, washing, and the administration of infant eye ointment. Left unhindered, healthy babies can find their mother's breast and begin breastfeeding without assistance. However, you can gently guide your baby to your breast for that first feeding if your baby seems ready.

CHAPTER FIVE

Avoiding Separation After Birth

"I felt pressured to send my baby
to the nursery after he was born."

—Linda

While working as a neonatal practitioner, sometimes I am asked to evaluate a baby's health in the hospital nursery. I remember one such call during the midnight hours of an overnight shift. On the way to the newborn nursery, I crossed the dimly lit hallways of the maternity floor. These sleepy hallways were in stark contrast to the bright lights and bustle of activity inside the newborn nursery.

Babies in bassinets were lined in rows as a nurse prepared to weigh each one on a digital scale. Meanwhile, a nurse's assistant was stocking the drawers beneath each bassinet with diapers and linen. Several of the babies waiting to be weighed were crying hysterically. The unit secretary was busy preparing paperwork for two more babies being admitted to this mix from the labor and delivery unit. Adding to the overall sense of chaos was an obstetrician who decided to perform a circumcision and was searching for a nurse to assist him in preparing his tiny patient for the procedure. Above the din of wailing babies, ringing telephones, and the banter of nursing staff, the radio on the desk was playing the hit song from the latest winner of *American Idol.*

David, the baby boy whom I was to evaluate, was lying beneath the radiant warmer. Shortly after birth, David had been transported to the newborn nursery as part of the hospital's admission protocol. This seemingly benign practice of being taken from his mother and sent to the nursery was stressful for baby David, and he began to cry. He continued to cry throughout the admission process, which involved measuring, monitoring, and multiple needle sticks. David cried so hard and for so long that it compromised his physical well-being. Meanwhile, David's mother, Linda, had been encouraged to catch up on her sleep since she had been awake and in labor most of the night.

David's nurse explained that he had been crying, and his vital signs were above the normal range. I turned off the heat lamp and began to gently examine him. With the lights off, David opened his blue eyes and began to gaze around. He made subtle mouth movements and turned his head from side to side, all signs that the six-hour-old baby was hungry and searching for his mother. Although his heart and respiratory rate were a bit elevated, he was otherwise perfectly normal. After reviewing David's birth record and finding nothing abnormal, I decided to return him to his mother.

David's mother, Linda, was awake when I knocked on her hospital room door. After introducing myself, I explained that the nurses had been concerned about her son's abnormal vital signs. I further explained that David's elevated vital signs were a symptom of stress and that what he needed more than anything was his mother. Linda was more than willing to help her son by holding him in the skin-to-skin position. A short while after placing them together, David began to breastfeed. Following an hour of close contact with his mother, David's vital signs returned to normal. No blood work, X-rays, or further testing were necessary.

WHAT IS SEPARATION?

Separation means that you and your baby are physically apart for a measurable amount of time. Separation may occur as the result of a legitimate medical need such as a premature infant being transferred to a neonatal intensive care unit. However, more often than not, a mother and her baby become separated because of routine hospital practices. This is what happened to Linda and baby David. A few hours after giving birth, Linda was transferred to her postpartum room, and David was sent to the nursery down the hall.

Sometimes it's not geographic distance that separates a mother from her baby. As we learned in Chapter Four, separation can occur while a mother and her baby are in the same room but are physically disconnected from each other. This type of separation occurs when a newborn is under the radiant warmer or is tightly swaddled instead of being held skin-to-skin.

WHY IS SEPARATION HARMFUL TO MY NEWBORN?

Let's take a closer look at what happened the night that baby David went to the newborn nursery. After birth, David spent a couple of hours in the delivery room where he was held by both of his parents. In the company of their familiar voices, he opened his eyes and briefly breastfed. When David was barely two hours old, he was placed in a bassinet and wheeled into the newborn nursery. Once inside the nursery, David's senses were assaulted by bright fluorescent lights and noises he had never heard before. Besides the unfamiliar voices of hospital staff, the nursery was full of buzzing alarms, ringing telephones, and crying babies. Unable to process this overwhelming mix of sensory stimulation, David began to cry.

After looking him over, David's nurse injected his thigh with a standard dose of vitamin K. This injection is traditionally given in the newborn period to prevent a rare bleeding syndrome. Vitamin K is produced in our intestines and is necessary to help blood properly clot. Since it takes about a week for a baby's body to produce its own vitamin K, the injection serves to fill the gap.

Next, David was washed with soap and water from head to toe. Although his nurse made quick work of this task, David cried the entire time. After his bath, he was put under the warmer where the heat would dry his wet hair, and the nurse could observe him. David had been crying for quite some time, and when his nurse placed him in his bassinet, she noticed that his arms were a bit jittery. Knowing that hypoglycemia or low blood sugar can cause a baby to exhibit such symptoms, she obtained a blood sample by sticking a lancet into the side of David's freshly washed foot. Thankfully, the glucometer registered David's blood sugar as within the normal range.

In response to the heel stick, David's already hard cry intensified. During this desperate bout of sustained crying, the nurse noticed that David's color had paled and that his heart rate had become abnormally high. After paging the pediatrician on call, the nurse requested that a NICU nurse practitioner come to the nursery to evaluate David.

David was born with a normal heart and lungs. However, his prolonged crying altered the otherwise normal function of his heart. David's excessive crying in reaction to an overstimulating environment, painful procedures, and separation from his mother caused his heart rate and blood pressure to significantly increase. This hard crying caused pressure changes in the right and left sides of his heart. These pressure changes allowed unoxygenated blood to circulate in his body. As a result, David's color changed and alarmed his nurse.

Following birth, a baby's heart and lungs undergo a series of miraculous changes. These changes allow a baby to adjust to life outside the mother's body. During this sensitive adjustment period, a newborn's cardiovascular system is vulnerable to stress, including the stress brought on by hard crying. Since the events that led to David's distress occurred during a period of routine separation, his parents were unable to comfort him. By the time I made my way to David's bedside, he had quieted down. He was almost too quiet. It was as if he had given up in total exhaustion.

ISN'T CRYING GOOD FOR MY NEWBORN?

Nearly everyone believes that it is beneficial for a newborn to cry after birth. However, research has shown that the birth cry is not necessary for adequate lung function.[1] Normal breathing provides a healthy baby with an adequate amount of air. Far from being beneficial, prolonged crying can be harmful to your newborn. Hard crying can cause abnormal elevations in your baby's heart rate and blood pressure that can compromise blood flow.[2] Additionally, continued crying causes your baby to swallow air, and this build up of air makes your baby more uncomfortable.[3]

These negative experiences can have a lasting effect on a baby.[4] Once a negative experience activates the stress response, it is quickly reactivated by any subsequent painful stimulation. For example, if a baby becomes distressed during multiple needle sticks, he or she will quickly exhibit the same intense stress reaction to an immunization given at a later date. Luckily, you can minimize the stress your baby experiences and eliminate unnecessary crying simply by being with your baby. It is a fact that babies who are held skin-to-skin after birth cry much less than babies in bassinets or under warmers.[5]

CAN I COMFORT MY NEWBORN DURING ROUTINE PROCEDURES?

Liza witnessed how upset her first baby became during the routine injections and lab tests that are part of hospital protocol. She described feeling helpless to comfort her son as he cried hysterically. Liza was determined to lessen the stress of routine hospital procedures after her second baby, Maya, was born. Liza planned to hold and breastfeed Maya instead of sending her to the nursery for these admission procedures.

At first, the nurse was hesitant to give Maya an injection and collect a blood sample from her heel while Maya was in her mother's arms. Eventually, the nurse agreed, and Liza said Maya hardly flinched during the needle sticks and continued to breastfeed. Liza, a pediatrician, now suggests that new mothers in her practice breastfeed their babies during routine immunizations.

Research supports what Liza and Maya discovered. Skin-to-skin holding and breastfeeding dramatically reduce the crying associated with painful procedures.[6] Babies who are held in skin-to-skin contact during painful procedures, even after surgery, cry much less than babies who are not held. Additionally, breastfeeding a baby can drastically reduce the pain and stress response to immunizations and blood tests.[7] The act of breastfeeding releases powerful hormones in your baby's body that function as natural painkillers. As you can see, breastfeeding is powerful medicine. Your newborn needs to be close to you to receive all that you have to offer as a mother.

CAN I SEND MY NEWBORN TO THE NURSERY AT NIGHT?

I was taught in nursing school that in order for a mother and her baby to sleep after childbirth, a mother must send her newborn to the nursery. During the daylight hours, a mother was expected to tend to her infant, but around midnight, the baby must enter the nurse's domain. As an Army nurse, I made this nursing school lesson part of my military mission. Once darkness settled outside the brick-walled hospital where I was stationed, I began to collect each baby from the maternity ward. After ordering the mothers to go immediately to sleep, I wheeled the long line of bassinets down the hall toward the nursery. Securely behind the nursery doors, I organized the individual bassinets according to Army standards. If someone happened to peer into the nursery windows while I was on duty, they would see rows of identically wrapped, precisely positioned newborns.

With all babies present and accounted for, I would turn my attention to collating data for the hospital's twenty-four-hour report. In short order, a high-ranking Army Nurse Corps officer would visit the nursery ward and collect my report. She, in turn, would reassemble the information in my report and report to the hospital commander. With so much reporting to do, nobody cared about breastfeeding.

That Army hospital closed years ago, but the belief that mothers and babies should be separated to sleep at night lives on. Studies show that new mothers in the hospital get roughly five hours of sleep whether their newborn is with them or not.[8] Regardless of this fact, the issue of sleeping after childbirth is of major concern to nearly every client I visit.

I remember one family whose breastfeeding troubles could be traced back to nighttime separation after birth. I met Natalie and her husband, Joe, several days after the birth of their daughter, Rosie. Natalie and Rosie were having difficulty connecting for feedings. When asked how their initial feedings went while in the hospital, Natalie said she had some success feeding Rosie during the day, but she hadn't been with Rosie at night until they arrived home from the hospital.

Each evening Joe returned home from the hospital to tend to the couple's two black labs, but before leaving the hospital each night, he would put Rosie in her bassinet and wheel her into the nursery so that Natalie could sleep. Once or twice during the course of the night, a nurse would bring Rosie to Natalie's room to breastfeed, but these feedings were seldom productive. Rosie was either crying frantically or in a deep sleep. As a result of repeated separation during the night, Natalie and Joe missed the opportunity to get acquainted with Rosie's signals of feeding readiness. While spending the night in the nursery, Rosie's subtle signals of hunger were most likely also missed. When she later awoke, Rosie was frantic with hunger, and by the time the nurses returned Rosie to Natalie's room, mother and daughter were out of sync.

My job in working with Natalie and Joe was to help them become familiar with Rosie's hunger signals. I also explained that young babies like

Rosie are hungrier at nighttime than during the day. In the initial period after birth, frequent nighttime feedings help a new mother to build a full milk supply. Sending Rosie to the nursery at night not only hindered her ability to become an effective breastfeeder; it could have had a negative impact on Natalie's future milk supply.

The hormones that help a new mother build a milk supply naturally peak during the nighttime hours.[9] This may be why young babies feel the urge to breastfeed at these times. The time and effort that you spend taking advantage of this natural phenomenon will be rewarded. You are literally investing in your future abundant milk supply. By learning to recognize and respond to Rosie's hunger signals, Natalie reported that feedings improved during the day as well as during the night. Now back in sync, Natalie and Rosie went on to develop a strong breastfeeding relationship.

HOW TO AVOID SEPARATION IN THE HOSPITAL

Use the following steps to avoid routine separation and related breastfeeding difficulty in the hospital.

Rest with your baby

You and your baby can recover together after birth. The best way to rest together is to hold your baby in the skin-to-skin position described in Chapter Four. Skin-to-skin holding benefits you, your newborn, and your breastfeeding relationship. The security of being held close to your body physically warms your newborn and prevents unnecessary crying. This effortless embrace affords you the opportunity to close your eyes and rest as a couple. As you do this, the hormone oxytocin begins circulating in your body, priming your milk flow. Oxytocin also has a positive influence on your emotions, naturally inducing a sense of well-being that helps you to fall in love with your new baby.[10] This simple act of resting with your baby lays the hormonal groundwork for your breastfeeding relationship.

Recognize feeding readiness

Staying together allows you the opportunity to recognize your newborn's first expressions of hunger. These hunger expressions can be very subtle and easily missed. When you miss your baby's early signals, you miss an opportunity to breastfeed while your newborn is relaxed. If these early signals go unheeded, a young baby will likely fall back to sleep. Eventually, a more potent sensation of hunger will cause your baby to wake up crying. *Crying is a sign of advanced hunger.* It is much more difficult to breastfeed a hungry frustrated newborn than one who is calm and alert. By keeping your new baby close, you can recognize these early signs of feeding readiness and make learning to breastfeed a positive experience for both of you. Common expressions of newborn hunger include the following:

- Head turning to one side
- Mouth opening and forming an "O" sign
- Hand going toward mouth
- Eyes opening and waking up

Recruit a hospital companion

If you are recovering from a cesarean section or a difficult birth, you will need assistance to avoid becoming separated from your baby. Someone will need to stay in your hospital room with you to assist with diaper changes and to help you position your baby for skin-to-skin holding. Any helpful friend or relative can serve as a hospital companion. A hospital companion would have helped my clients Natalie and Joe. If you remember, each evening, Joe returned home to care for their dogs, leaving Natalie in her hospital room and baby Rosie in the nursery for the night. To foster Natalie's breastfeeding relationship with Rosie, perhaps a friend could have stayed in Natalie's hospital room so that Rosie could spend the night close to her mother. In the interest of avoiding separation, an alternative solution would have been to ask a friend to dog-sit so that Joe could spend the night with his family.

Request that all procedures be done in your room

Having all newborn admission procedures done in your room instead of in the hospital nursery will enable you to quickly comfort your baby with skin-to-skin holding and breastfeeding. After a stressful procedure, breastfeeding will continue to comfort your baby. Of all the hospital practices that traditionally make up the newborn admission process, the one that produces the most angst is the sponge bath. I have witnessed babies just a few hours old cry so furiously while being rubbed clean with a wet washcloth that their entire body turns bright red. A more compassionate alternative would be a full body bath in a small tub of warm water. Unfortunately, our cultural obsession over keeping a newborn's umbilical cord stump bone dry immediately after birth prohibits this practice.

Research has demonstrated that skin-to-skin holding and breastfeeding have a powerful analgesic effect on your newborn, dramatically reducing the pain of injections and blood draws. Breastfeeding during a procedure works best if you first take the time to get your baby well attached to your breast. Once both of you are settled, and you feel the tugging sensation of active sucking, the nurse can administer the injection or draw blood from your baby. If your baby detaches from your breast during the procedure, help your baby reattach.

SUMMARY OF BREASTFEEDING ABCs

After giving birth, there are many benefits to keeping your newborn next to you both day and night. Being with you naturally calms your baby during hospital admission procedures. With fewer bouts of crying, your baby will be better able to breastfeed. Keeping your baby with you in your hospital room provides you with the opportunity to recognize your baby's early hunger signals. Beginning to breastfeed when your baby is ready makes learning to nurse a positive experience. These frequent feedings serve to establish your milk supply and will benefit your future breastfeeding relationship.

A. ADMISSION

Ask that all newborn admission procedures be conducted in your hospital room instead of in the newborn nursery. This way you will avoid becoming separated from your baby for a long period of time. If your baby becomes upset during the admission process, you can provide comfort by holding, touching, and talking to your baby. With your baby in your room, you can observe your baby's signs of feeding readiness. It is common for newborns to breastfeed frequently throughout the night. This helps your baby to become an established breastfeeder and it helps to stimulate your milk supply.

B. BEGIN

Begin breastfeeding when your baby shows signs of feeding readiness. It will always be easier to breastfeed when your baby is in the early stages of hunger. This is especially true after birth when you and your baby are learning together. Become familiar with your baby's unique way of expressing hunger. Classic signs of early hunger include your baby's head turning to one side, a wide-open mouth, or your baby bringing one or both hands toward his or her mouth.

C. COMFORT

Comfort your baby with skin-to-skin contact and breastfeeding. Contrary to common belief, crying does not promote aeration of your baby's lungs.

You can prevent excessive crying by breastfeeding your baby during potentially painful procedures. To do this, make sure your baby is comfortably attached to your breast and sucking before the injection or needle stick is given. Continue to comfort your baby with skin-to-skin holding and breastfeeding after the procedure is complete.

CHAPTER SIX

Bottle and Breast:
Preventing Feeding Confusion

"I wish my baby had never been given a bottle."

—Paula

When first born, baby Emily was breastfeeding beautifully. However, four days later her mother, Paula, developed complications related to her cesarean section that necessitated a return to the operating room. During the surgery and recovery period, Emily was in the newborn nursery, where she was bottle-fed by the nurses. When mother and daughter were reunited, Emily was unable to breastfeed. In the weeks that followed, Paula used an electric breast pump while trying to get Emily back to breast. Unfortunately, Paula's milk supply dwindled, and nothing seemed to work.

With a few simple adjustments, this story could have had a more positive outcome. Paula was not aware that giving bottles to a baby Emily's age could confuse her and put their future as a breastfeeding couple at risk. If Paula had this information, she could have requested that Emily be temporarily fed by an alternative method that supports breastfeeding such as finger feeding or cup feeding. Once Paula was healthy, Emily could have resumed breastfeeding without the risk of feeding confusion.

WHAT IS FEEDING CONFUSION?

I use the term *feeding confusion* to describe what happens when a baby is unable to effectively breastfeed after bottle-feeding or pacifier sucking. In the initial days after birth, a baby's mouth is acutely sensitive to any stimulation. A pacifier, bottle, or sucking on your finger stimulates your baby's mouth differently than your nipple. A newborn can easily become accustomed to this overstimulation of the tongue and hard palate. Once accustomed to the sensation of a bottle or pacifier, your baby will have difficulty readjusting his or her tongue position to effectively breastfeed. Feeding confusion can occur after just one exposure to a bottle or pacifier.

Whenever I hear the term *nipple confusion,* I am reminded of a scene in the movie *Meet the Fockers.* In the movie, Robert De Niro plays a grandfather who "feeds" his grandson pumped breast milk from a prosthetic breast to prevent the baby from developing nipple confusion while his mother is away. Upon meeting the grandfather, Barbra Streisand's character enquires, "You are preventing confusion by strapping a boob on a man?" Of course, nipple confusion is not so humorous for my clients who are experiencing breastfeeding difficulty. Instead of *nipple confusion,* I use the term *feeding confusion* to describe what happens when a baby is unable to breastfeed following some other oral experience.

As was the case with my client Paula and her baby, Emily, feeding confusion occurred after Emily successfully breastfed and was subsequently given bottles. Sometimes feeding confusion results from a delay in the establishment of the breastfeeding relationship, and a young baby who has never breastfed becomes accustomed to an alternate way of feeding. Ironically, it may be the same internal mechanism that is responsible for a newborn's urge to gravitate toward his or her mother's breast that predisposes newborns to developing feeding confusion.

According to the "imprinting" theory, a newborn will form an attachment to anything that is introduced into its mouth and will quickly develop a strong preference to a particular feeding modality.[1] This is especially true during the first few days of life when a baby's mouth is acutely sensitive to the sensations that accompany the feeling of being fed. A baby will quickly form a habit of holding his or her tongue in a certain way to receive a feeding. In baby Emily's situation, she became accustomed to the overstimulation that the bottle nipple provided to the roof of her mouth. After multiple bottle feedings, she was unable to remember how to attach to her mother's nipple. When brought to Paula's breast, Emily would either cry in frustration or fall asleep. When she was hungry, Emily expected and responded to the sensation of the bottle nipple in her mouth and not her mother's nipple.

THE PROBLEM WITH PACIFIERS

I believe a pacifier can confuse both of you! Maryellen's story illustrates how a pacifier confuses a mother's ability to interpret her newborn's hunger signals as it interferes with a baby's ability to communicate hunger. Maryellen asked to see me after her daughter Larissa's two-week appointment with the pediatrician. Larissa was still several ounces below her birth weight, and the doctor told Maryellen that she needed to supplement Larissa with formula. The following morning, I went to see Maryellen and Larissa in their home.

Maryellen welcomed me into her comfortable living room. As I set up my scale, Maryellen described Larissa as a quiet baby who rarely cried and had to be awakened for breastfeeding. In fact, as we spoke Larissa was still upstairs asleep in her crib. When I met Larissa, she appeared drowsy but had a firm grip on the pacifier in her mouth. I quickly got the sense that pacifier sucking was the culprit of this couple's breastfeeding difficulty. Maryellen explained that she was exhausted after giving birth and had given Larissa a pacifier hoping that it would help Larissa to sleep longer. As the days passed, Larissa sucked on her pacifier more and more often. If the pacifier slipped from her mouth, Maryellen and her husband fell into the habit of pushing it back into Larissa's mouth.

Constant sucking camouflaged Larissa's subtle hunger cues. Unable to recognize when Larissa was hungry, Maryellen began to schedule and time Larissa's feedings. Meanwhile, Larissa's mouth became accustomed to the strong sensation of a stiff pacifier nipple, and her breastfeeding skills suffered. I explained to Maryellen that breastfeeding was not the problem, rather the pacifier was to blame for Larissa's slow weight gain. Pacifier sucking had replaced precious opportunities to breastfeed.

Sure enough, a few minutes after Maryellen removed the pacifier from Larissa's mouth and held her in the skin-to-skin position, she began to make recognizable hunger signals. Together, we assisted Larissa to comfortably attach to her mother's breast. Maryellen soon realized that when Larissa opened her lips and moved her hands toward her mouth, she needed her mother's milk, not her pacifier. Over the next week, Maryellen and Larissa breastfed often and took a break from the pacifier. At her follow-up visit, Maryellen was proud to see that Larissa had gained back her birth weight. Just as important, Maryellen and Larissa had found their way back together as a breastfeeding couple.

Sometimes chronic pacifier use signals a painful problem in the breastfeeding relationship.[2] This was the case with Sydney and her fifth child, Milo. Having successfully breastfed four other children, Sydney knew that breastfeeding should not be painful. A few days after arriving home from the hospital with Milo, Sydney found breastfeeding unbearable and began giving Milo a pacifier to avoid the pain of frequent feedings. Sydney found that the pacifier lengthened the time between Milo's feedings and gave her a chance to cope with the demands of caring for her large family. Unfortunately, ten days later, Sydney's nipple pain had not improved; in fact, it was worse.

Nipple candidiasis was the likely cause of the burning and stinging pain that Sydney described. This condition is usually easy to treat, and during our consultation, I prescribed the appropriate ointments. Pacifiers can serve as vectors for yeast and bacteria, exacerbating an already painful condition by passing it back and forth between mother and infant.[3] Once she was comfortable, Sydney breastfed Milo more often and used the pacifier less. Mothering four young children and a newborn is a tall task for anyone, but Sydney seemed to take it all in stride.

IS IT EVER OKAY TO USE A PACIFIER?

As we discussed, pacifiers are not without risk. Offered after birth, they can lead to dysfunctional and ineffective breastfeeding.[4] Chronic pacifier sucking can potentially disrupt the development of your breastfeeding relationship by masking your newborn's hunger signals and causing your newborn to miss valuable time at your breast. Pacifiers can easily become colonized with yeast and bacteria, increasing the spread of nipple infections. However, in certain circumstances, a pacifier can be useful. For instance, sucking eases the pain a baby experiences during medical procedures.[5] Aside from isolated use, if you feel compelled to have your baby suck a pacifier then first allow your breastfeeding relationship to grow and bloom without the interference of artificial nipples. Once you have an established milk supply and are breastfeeding comfortably, a pacifier is less likely to disturb the natural rhythm of your relationship.

There will be many times when your baby signals a need to be close to you. Breastfeeding your baby at these times is just as important as the feedings that provide a calorie-dense meal. Part of what makes breastfeeding a truly complex relationship is that it cannot be fully quantified. The mysterious nature of a harmonious breastfeeding relationship cannot be weighed, measured, or plotted like scientific data on a graph. Breastfeeding nourishes your baby's body and comforts your baby's soul. In fact, the German word for breastfeeding is *stillen,* which is translated as "to quiet and comfort," which I believe more fully describes the multifaceted nature of the breastfeeding relationship.

IS MY COLOSTRUM ENOUGH?

Bradley was a healthy baby boy, born weighing eight pounds eight ounces. After birth, he was initially sleepy, but then he regularly woke for feedings and made several wet and meconium diapers. When Bradley was forty-eight hours old, he was reweighed and the night nurse told Bradley's mother, Lisa, that he now weighed eight pounds one ounce. Lisa was so upset by the news that Bradley has lost seven ounces that she immediately fed him two ounces of formula from a hospital bottle. Lisa had thought that breastfeeding was going well, but now she believed that Bradley was not getting enough nourishment.

Although Lisa was alarmed by the news that Bradley weighed less at two days of age than at birth, Bradley's weight loss is part of a normal process called *contraction*. Babies born near their due dates are naturally equipped with extra fat and fluid that are meant to be metabolized in the first days of life. Far from failing to nourish her son, Lisa's colostrum was hard at work protecting Bradley from illness as well as priming and preparing his body for the supply of mature milk that was on its way. In fact, the large meconium stools Bradley passed resulted from the laxative effect of colostral milk on his intestines. These stools accounted for part of his weight loss.

The following afternoon as Lisa was getting ready to leave the hospital her breasts became full and warm, a sure sign that her mature milk had arrived right on schedule. Like many new mothers, Lisa had become understandably frightened by the news of her newborn's initial weight loss and reacted by feeding him formula that he did not need. Healthy babies like Bradley do not need sterile water, sugar water, or formula.

Supplemental feedings are often more harmful than helpful. Sterile water and sugar water have no nutritional value and take up precious space in a newborn's tiny stomach. This feeling of fullness leads to a missed opportunity to breastfeed and a missed opportunity to receive the benefits of colostrum. Formula is not benign either. Even one formula feeding like

Bradley received alters the delicate chemistry inside a newborn's intestines.[6] Early exposure to the cow's milk or soy ingredients in standard formula can predispose a newborn to developing a food allergy later in childhood.[7] Supplementation with bottles of formula may predispose breastfeeding babies and their mothers to becoming infected with candidiasis.[8]

Initial feedings of colostrum are designed to be small in volume but high in nutritional and immunologic value. Unfortunately, the fast flow of a bottle can force a newborn like Bradley to gulp a much larger amount of formula than is physiologically appropriate. Once ingested, formula forms a hard curd in a baby's digestive tract, leading to constipation. In the interest of protecting a newborn's digestive system and a mother's developing milk supply, supplemental feedings are not recommended by the World Health Organization or the American Academy of Pediatrics unless medically indicated.

WHEN IS A SUPPLEMENT NECESSARY?

Healthy babies born close to their due date do not need to be fed water or formula. Besides being unavoidably separated from your newborn for an extended period of time, there are a few situations that sometimes warrant supplemental feedings. In each of the four situations outlined next, the preferable supplement is always your own pumped colostrum or breast milk. Because colostrum is thick, it can be difficult to pump, so sometimes hand expression works better.

Besides your breast milk, the next best supplement is donated breast milk. Breast milk from a human milk bank is collected from mothers in good health who donate their surplus supply of pumped frozen breast milk. The milk bank then thaws and combines the milk from several women. The pooled milk is then pasteurized and refrozen for distribution. Much of the donated milk goes to hospitals to use in their neonatal intensive care units, but I have had clients purchase donor milk for an adopted baby. The down side of donor milk from a milk bank is that it is very expensive. From time to time, I have clients who wish to give their surplus supply of breast milk to another mother or who accept breast milk from a friend or family member. Before sharing breast milk, it is important to be sure that the milk donor is HIV negative because the virus that causes AIDS can live in breast milk.[9] Since breast milk changes as your baby matures, it is preferable if the milk donor's baby is nearly the same age as the recipient's baby. If you are unable to pump your milk or obtain donated breast milk, then the last choice is a formula supplement.

Low blood sugar

The medical term for low blood sugar is *hypoglycemia*. Infants whose mothers are diabetic or develop diabetes during pregnancy may be at risk for having low blood sugar after birth. Very small or very large newborns can also become hypoglycemic. Symptoms of hypoglycemia include jitteriness. A simple blood test can determine if a baby's blood sugar is low. It is important to treat hypoglycemia because a baby's brain depends on glucose to function properly. Breastfeeding soon after birth is especially important if your newborn is at risk for hypoglycemia. Besides frequent breastfeeding, the treatment for hypoglycemia includes supplemental feedings and possibly IV fluids until normal blood sugar levels are achieved.

Jaundice

A few days after birth, it is common for a newborn's skin to become yellow or jaundice in color. The medical term for this condition is *hyperbilirubinemia*. Jaundice occurs when red blood cells break down, and the by-products of the red cells called *bilirubin* accumulate before being processed by the liver. Mild or moderate jaundice is considered physiologic and will resolve naturally. Factors such as blood type incompatibility, prematurity, or illness can cause bilirubin levels to rise above physiologic levels, thereby necessitating treatment with phototherapy lights and IV fluids.

Cessation of breastfeeding is not necessary because the laxative effect of breast milk helps your baby to excrete bilirubin by stooling.

Excessive weight loss

As discussed earlier in this chapter, all newborns lose some weight after birth. It can be normal for a baby to lose up to 7 percent of his or her birth weight.[10] For example, a baby born weighing seven pounds may lose up to eight ounces before the loss is considered problematic. Frequent feedings of colostrum prevent excessive weight loss and prepare your baby for the arrival of your mature milk. Keeping your baby close and holding your baby in the skin-to-skin position will encourage frequent breastfeeding. A lack of wet and meconium stool diapers can be a signal that your newborn is not breastfeeding effectively or frequently enough. Excessive weight loss signals a problem in the breastfeeding relationship that needs to be remedied. Supplementing may be necessary as you work toward a solution.

Delayed onset of mature milk

Sometimes a newborn's excessive weight loss can be the result of a delay in the onset of a mother's mature breast milk. Most mothers remember the arrival of their mature milk because their breasts become very full, firm, and warm. This is called *primary engorgement* and usually occurs around the third or fourth day after birth. At this time, the smaller amounts of yellow colostrum give way to a larger volume of white breast milk. Several factors can cause a delay in the arrival of a mother's abundant milk supply. Having a difficult birth, an unplanned cesarean section, or a very large baby can cause a delay in primary engorgement.[11] Some medical conditions such as diabetes, hormonal imbalances, or obesity have also been shown to affect a mother's milk supply. If you are at risk for delayed milk production, supplemental feedings may be necessary. Keep in mind that many mothers who are at risk for delayed primary engorgement make copious amounts of mature milk right on schedule!

WILL SUPPLEMENTING HURT BREASTFEEDING?

Your breastfeeding relationship is not doomed if you are faced with a situation that requires supplemental feeding. If your baby needs a supplement, choose a plan that supports breastfeeding. My client Nancy faced this situation when her son Ben was born four weeks before he was expected. Luckily, Ben was healthy and began breastfeeding soon after birth. But by two days of age, Ben became jaundiced. Because Ben was born a bit early, the doctor recommended phototherapy and supplemental formula feeding.

Although the phototherapy lamp would lower Ben's rising bilirubin level, it would increase his needs for fluids. For this reason, supplemental feedings or IV fluids, in addition to breastfeeding, are often part of the treatment for hyperbilirubinemia. Because of a history of food allergies in the family, Nancy wanted to avoid supplementing Ben with formula. I recommended that she begin pumping with one of the hospital's double electric breast pumps. Because Ben was Nancy's second baby, I predicted that she would make plenty of breast milk. Experienced mothers can expect their mature milk to come in sooner and in greater volume than a first-time mother. Sure enough, Nancy did express enough milk to give to Ben as a supplement. In order to avoid feeding confusion, Nancy requested that her pumped breast milk be fed to Ben with a syringe instead of a bottle, and she continued to breastfeed him during his allotted breaks from phototherapy. Ben responded well to this treatment plan, and soon he was discharged from the hospital. At home, he continued to breastfeed without confusion.

Nancy had the advantage of being an experienced mother with an abundant milk supply. This enabled her to use her own pumped milk as a supplement instead of formula. This was not the case for Jill, who wanted to breastfeed her son Zachary but had had breast reduction surgery three years prior to giving birth. When I met Jill, baby Zachary was one week old and a full pound below his birth weight. He was sleeping most of the time, and I knew he needed the volume and calories of supplemental feedings.

Throughout her pregnancy, Jill had looked forward to breastfeeding her baby. I assured Jill that she could share a breastfeeding relationship with Zachary. However, Zachary needed much more milk than she was physically able to produce. During our consultation, I taught Jill to supplement Zachary with formula as he breastfed by using a supplemental nursing system (SNS). The SNS consists of a bottle and a set of thin flexible tubing. The bottle fits around a mother's neck like an adjustable necklace and the tubing is taped to her breast. During a feeding a baby attaches to the breast as well as the tubing so that the baby receives both the contents of the bottle through the tubing and the milk from the breast. This device enabled Zachary to receive a supplemental feeding of formula while simultaneously receiving Jill's milk from her breast. Jill was highly motivated and tireless in her effort to make the most of her milk supply. Besides using the SNS, Jill began pumping with a hospital-grade breast pump at regular intervals, and she began taking a prescription drug to stimulate her milk supply. As time passed, Zachary grew and Jill reached her goal of being able to breastfeed Zachary for several feedings a day without an additional supplement. Best of all, Jill told me, "Zachary loves breastfeeding as much as I do."

Breast reduction surgery affects a mother's ability to produce a full milk supply because breast tissue that could potentially make breast milk is removed and nerves around the nipple are injured when it is repositioned over the reshaped breast.[12] When breastfeeding after breast reduction surgery, I recommend supplementing your baby early to prevent excessive weight loss. I have worked with many mothers who breastfeed after breast reduction surgery, and the best way to supplement is to use the SNS like Jill did. When breastfeeding after reduction surgery, the overall goal is not merely milk production but the enjoyment of the entire breastfeeding experience.

HOW DO I AVOID FEEDING CONFUSION IF I NEED TO SUPPLEMENT?

Nancy and Jill had legitimate reasons to give supplemental feedings to their newborns. Both mothers chose to supplement in a breastfeeding-friendly manner that preserved the future of their breastfeeding relationship. Remember, most babies do not need supplemental feedings; however, if your newborn does require supplements, use the following steps as a guide to avoid feeding confusion.

Protect you baby's palate

Your newborn's mouth is very sensitive. Avoid introducing anything into your baby's mouth until breastfeeding is well established. The sensation of a stiff pacifier or bottle nipple can interfere with your baby's ability to cultivate an effective breastfeeding suck.

Promote frequent feeding

Many of the situations that necessitate supplementation can be avoided altogether by frequent breastfeeding after birth, which helps to prevent excessive weight loss, low blood sugar, and jaundice. Holding your baby in skin-to-skin contact encourages your baby to breastfeed frequently and to receive the benefits of your colostrum. Frequent breastfeeding will help you to establish a full milk supply.

Pick breastfeeding-friendly alternatives

When faced with a situation that requires supplementing, always pick the solution that most supports breastfeeding. This means supplementing with your pumped colostrum or breast milk if possible. If your baby is attaching to your breast but needs more volume, then use an SNS device. If your baby is unable to effectively attach to your breast or if you become unavoidably separated, consider a syringe, a dropper, or cup feeding. These are temporary measures, and the idea is to return your baby to your breast as soon as possible. If after several days of supplementing your baby is still unable to attach to your breast, consider trying a nipple shield. Used correctly and at the appropriate time, a nipple shield can help to bridge the gap between supplemental feeding and breastfeeding.

SUMMARY OF BREASTFEEDING ABCs

I use the term *feeding confusion* instead of *nipple confusion* to describe what happens when a young baby is unable to effectively breastfeed following some other oral experience. A bottle or pacifier overstimulates your newborn's sensitive mouth. A newborn can easily become accustomed to this hyperstimulation and have difficulty breastfeeding afterward. Most babies do not need water or formula, but if you have to supplement, try first to use your pumped colostrum or breast milk. Remember, the idea is to resume breastfeeding as soon as possible.

A. ALTERNATIVES

If your newborn requires supplemental feeding, choose a breastfeeding-friendly alternative. Providing a supplement by dropper, syringe, or cup will go a long way in preventing feeding confusion that can occur after exposure to a bottle nipple. Bottle nipples and pacifiers overstimulate your baby's mouth and can interfere with your baby's ability to effectively breastfeed.

B. BEGIN

Begin breastfeeding as soon as possible after birth. In many cases, early feeding can prevent the need for supplements. By design, colostrum is small in volume but high in value and can help to prevent situations that require supplements. Holding your baby in skin-to-skin contact and keeping your baby in your hospital room instead of the nursery will make these early feedings easier.

C. COLOSTRUM

Your colostrum is full of living cells that protect your newborn from illness. Your colostral milk is available to your baby immediately after birth even if your baby is born earlier than expected. Colostrum is meant to prepare your baby's stomach and intestines for the arrival of mature breast milk. It is normal for your newborn to lose some weight after birth. When your baby is about four days old, your higher-volume breast milk will arrive, and your baby will begin to grow and gain weight.

Phase II

Beginning to Breastfeed Your Baby

The time that follows the birth of your baby is a time like no other; not only filled with great excitement, these first weeks of your baby's life can be overwhelming. In my private practice as a lactation consultant, I have worked with hundreds of new mothers as they simultaneously recover from giving birth and adjust to their new life as a breastfeeding mother. Navigating through this transition can be difficult. These next five chapters address the very issues that have challenged my clients. Knowing when to breastfeed your baby, knowing how to position yourself comfortably while breastfeeding, and knowing what's important to keep track of will help make beginning to breastfeed a positive experience. This is also the ideal time to become familiar with common breastfeeding problems so that you can recognize when to seek the assistance of a professional lactation consultant.

CHAPTER SEVEN

The Signals That Will Let You Know When to Feed Your Baby

"I can't tell when my baby is hungry."

—JENNIFER

After ten years as a school guidance counselor, Jennifer felt ready to have a child of her own. Jennifer was accustomed to a busy workday; she took pride in her neatly organized office and always finished her reports before they were due. However, when Jennifer arrived home from the hospital with baby Elise, Jennifer entered an unfamiliar world of around-the-clock motherhood. As a new mother, she felt her work was never done. Elise seemed to need her all day and all night! There was barely enough time to shower let alone enjoy an afternoon coffee break. Jennifer was feeling overwhelmed when a girlfriend gave her a book that recommended mothers establish a strict schedule when feeding their babies. Jennifer decided to give it a try and began breastfeeding Elise every three hours and putting her in a crib for prescribed naps. Elise protested this regimen with fits of hysterical crying, especially when left alone in her crib. When offered one of her scheduled feedings, Elise was often too upset to breastfeed effectively. After a few days of this misery, Jennifer wasn't sure if it was breastfeeding or the new schedule that wasn't working.

It's easy to sympathize with Jennifer's frustration. As a professional goal-oriented woman, Jennifer was accustomed to being organized and finishing one task before beginning another. When Jennifer arrived home from the hospital with Elise, she may have had an easier time navigating the uncharted waters of new motherhood had she known that it takes time for mothers, babies, and breastfeeding to fall in sync. It is common for a new mother and her baby to experience an initial period of ambiguity, even chaos, as they become accustomed to each other. Thankfully, this period of confusion is self-limiting, and most mothers and babies fall seamlessly into step. This natural pattern of compatibility emerges over time, not overnight. Establishing a breastfeeding relationship takes patience and perseverance. Eventually, you and your baby will develop a unique pattern of feeding, resting, and sleeping. As Jennifer discovered, this natural rhythm becomes stifled when an artificial schedule is superimposed over the needs of you and your baby.

HOW DO WE BECOME A BREASTFEEDING TEAM?

The first few weeks are a time of exploration and adjustment as you and your baby become acquainted. Some mothers just seem to have an easier time accepting this ambiguity. Tia is an example of such a mother. I met Tia when her daughter Sasha was a week old. During our consultation, Sasha breastfed well, and Tia asked lots of questions about breastfeeding and baby care.

What impressed me most about Tia was her ability to appreciate the ambiguity of new motherhood. She was able to tolerate the lack of absolute answers during this transition time and allow the process of breastfeeding Sasha to unfold. "Sasha and I are getting breastfeeding started by spending lots of time relaxing together. I don't want to make any big plans until we get this figured out." During this time, Tia didn't over organize her day or try to overanalyze Sasha's developing feeding and sleeping patterns. Rather, Tia spent time with Sasha and learned to recognize her hunger signals. As our visit drew to a close, I assured Tia that she would soon notice Sasha's natural pattern of feeding and sleeping.

Months later, I ran into Tia and Sasha on a shopping excursion. As Tia and I talked, Sasha gave me a big bright toothless smile. Rather than a difficult chore, Tia described breastfeeding as an effortless pleasure. She was now able to anticipate Sasha's hunger and noticed that her breasts became full of milk before feeding time. This connection continued even at night, and Tia would awaken a few moments before Sasha stirred in hunger. Tia happily remarked, "Sasha and I are a team!" As we said good-bye and I watched Tia walk away with Sasha in her arms, I couldn't help but think that they were much more than teammates. Tia and Sasha were true companions. This type of harmony can't be scheduled.

Tia was able to cultivate a high level of confidence in her ability to mother Sasha by giving herself time to get to know Sasha after she was born. Over time, she became adept at recognizing and responding to Sasha's signals. Sasha grew into a calm, friendly baby who thoroughly trusted Tia. Together, mother and daughter shared a rhythmic cycle of breastfeeding, satiety, and sleeping. Tia and Sasha's unique pattern for success cannot be scheduled.

CAN I SCHEDULE BREASTFEEDING?

I enjoy wonderful working relationships with nearly every family that I meet, and over the years a few clients have become close friends. It is rare that I meet someone with whom I am unable to forge a bond. Not only was I unable to connect with Rochelle personally but I was unable to help her professionally because her style of mothering was not conducive to breastfeeding.

I met Rochelle after she was discharged from the hospital with her second son, Justin. Rochelle was having trouble getting breastfeeding started. The fact that Justin was smaller than her first baby and born by an unplanned cesarean section could explain Rochelle's difficulty, but it was her allegiance to strict scheduling that was to blame for her breastfeeding troubles. When I arrived for our appointment, Rochelle informed me that she intended to train Justin to follow the same prescribed feeding and sleeping regimen that she instituted with her two-year-old son when he was a baby. Not wanting to waste any time, Rochelle had already begun indoctrinating five-day-old Justin to the plan.

As Rochelle spoke, Justin began to stir, and his tiny fingers were making their way toward his open mouth. I gently interrupted Rochelle and pointed out Justin's hunger signals and suggested that now would be an excellent time to begin breastfeeding. Rochelle balked and insisted on postponing the feeding until the scheduled time. For the remainder of the visit, I did my best to help Rochelle and Justin connect, but I felt my effort was futile. In the end, Rochelle placed her schedule above the needs of her infant son. After that visit, I did not hear from Rochelle again.

Babies respond to their inner sensations of hunger and experience stress when their hunger is not satisfied. Strict feeding schedules satisfy an adult's need for complete control over the process of parenting, but schedules do not satisfy an infant's need to be nurtured. Because breastfeeding is built on mutual trust, feeding schedules sabotage breastfeeding success. Rochelle obtained her schedule from a popular book, but many of my clients get similar scheduling advice from their pediatrician.

Lori had been exclusively breastfeeding her daughter Charlotte since birth. From early on, their breastfeeding relationship had been smooth and trouble-free. Lori had an abundant milk supply, and Charlotte was healthy and energetic. All was well until Lori took Charlotte to the pediatrician for a routine visit.

The pediatrician advised Lori to schedule Charlotte's feedings at three-hour intervals throughout the day. Over the preceding months, Lori and Charlotte had developed their own routine, which included multiple feedings especially in the late afternoon and evening. Most nights, Charlotte awakened to breastfeed and would quickly fall back to sleep. The pediatrician objected to these late-night feedings and stated that a baby Charlotte's age should not be fed during the night. After a few nights of crying, she would forget all about breastfeeding.

After returning home from the pediatrician's office, Lori's self-confidence was shaken. She was unsure about what to do and wanted to know what I thought about the doctor's regimen. I listened to Lori's concerns and then responded by asking Lori what she thought about the pediatrician's feeding schedule. After all, as Charlotte's mother, Lori was the expert. Nobody knows a baby better than the baby's own mother! Lori thought for a moment and replied that the restrictive schedule would make both of them miserable. Charlotte would cry in hunger, and Lori would be heartbroken hearing her daughter's desperate cries.

Although rigid feeding and sleeping schedules are still recommended by some doctors and nurses, they are based on formula-feeding guidelines not breastfeeding physiology. A newborn's stomach is about the size of his or her fist and designed for small frequent meals. These frequent feedings, especially during the night, serve to build a new mother's milk supply.[1] Limiting a baby's feedings can suppress a new mother's milk supply and cause a healthy baby to cry with hunger.

SHOULD I BREASTFEED ON DEMAND?

Another popular school of thought dictates that new mothers feed their baby on demand instead of on a schedule. The inherent negativity implied by "demand" feed lingo makes me cringe nearly as much as baby-care schedules. A baby should never need to cry out in hunger, demanding to be fed. Additionally distasteful is the assumption that a mother is passively waiting around in servitude to the whims of her baby. In a breastfeeding relationship, a mother is neither a dictator nor a wallflower.

A mother actively participates in the development of a baby's feeding and sleeping pattern. For instance, Jamie planned to work from home and wanted to be fully available for a daily conference call between 11 A.M. and noon. She purposely breastfed her daughter Lexie around ten thirty each morning so that Lexie would be satiated by 11 A.M., allowing Jamie to telecommute without interruption.

As you and your baby develop a unique pattern of daily life, notice your body's natural rhythm. If your breasts feel full of milk at a certain time each day, take advantage of your natural abundance by awakening your baby to breastfeed. It is important to remember that this daily pattern of hunger, feeding, and sleeping won't become recognizable until after the arrival of your mature milk and your baby's return to birth weight. To assure that this happens by two weeks of age, encourage your newborn to breastfeed frequently during the day as well as during the night.

HOW LONG SHOULD A FEEDING TAKE?

When I went to visit Jessica for a consultation, she seemed to have everything in order. Jessica had an excellent supply of milk, and her son, Coby, was gaining weight well. Yet, Jessica was worried that something was wrong with the way Coby was breastfeeding because he often breastfed for longer than ten minutes. Jessica's doctor had told her that after ten minutes her breasts were empty and that Coby "was using her as a pacifier." Like Jessica, almost all of my clients are concerned about the length of a feeding.

Contrary to what Jessica had been told, her breast was not completely empty after a specific number of minutes.[2] Because Jessica had cultivated a full milk supply, some breast milk was always available for Coby. She was relieved to learn that the high-fat milk Coby received near the end of a feeding, often referred to as *hind milk,* would help Coby to feel contented and promote his growth. Knowing that her breasts were never completely empty and that Coby's longer feeding style was normal enabled Jessica to relax and observe Coby instead of counting the passing minutes.

SHOULD MY BABY BREASTFEED FREQUENTLY AT NIGHT?

Betty was excited to become a grandmother for the first time. After her granddaughter, Avianna, was born, Betty dedicated herself to helping her daughter Jenna care for Avianna. When it came to breastfeeding, Betty felt at a loss because she had not breastfed. She was concerned that her granddaughter, Avianna, was breastfeeding too frequently during the night and interrupting Jenna's sleep. Based on her own experience as a formula-feeding mother, Betty advised her daughter to feed Avianna bottles of formula during the night instead of breastfeeding. Betty believed this would encourage her granddaughter to sleep through the night.

Betty's expectation that young babies should sleep for long blocks of time at night is based on a formula-feeding paradigm and not on breastfeeding physiology. Betty's well-intentioned plan would harm the development of Jenna's breastfeeding relationship with Avianna. It is, in fact, normal for Avianna to breastfeed frequently during the night. Contrary to what Betty thought, a young healthy baby like Avianna will be more awake during the night than during the day, and Avianna's frequent night-time feedings will help Jenna to establish a strong milk supply. By substituting formula at night instead of breastfeeding, Jenna's milk supply will quickly dwindle. As Avianna grows and time passes, she will naturally sleep longer at night and spend more time awake during the day. Certainly, Jenna could gently help Avianna adjust her feeding and sleeping patterns by offering extra breastfeeding sessions during the day.

HOW DO I KNOW IF A FEEDING IS PRODUCTIVE?

The passage of time does not gauge the success of breastfeeding. However, what happens during that time is very significant. Sometimes your baby may feed very effectively and receive a full feeding in just a few minutes. At other times, your baby may take longer to feel full and actively breastfeed for forty-five minutes. The same is true for the interval of time between feed-ings. During a feeding cluster, your baby may need to breastfeed every hour; at other times, your baby may not feel hungry for several hours. Timed feedings and prefabricated schedules cannot be trusted to gauge the overall health of your breastfeeding relationship. Instead of focusing on the passage of time, I recommend mothers learn to recognize three separate factors, which, when combined, serve to gauge the status of their breastfeeding re-lationship. Once your mature milk has arrived, learn to recognize your baby's feeding signals, diaper output, and feeding clusters as indicators that breastfeeding is progressing in a positive direction.

Recognize feeding signals

Rather than obsessing over the passage of time, become aware of what your baby is telling you during a feeding. By becoming alert, you can easily rec-ognize the signs of a productive feeding. Learn to look at your baby, listen to your baby, and feel what is happening during the feeding.

What to look for: As you'll see in the next chapter, a feeding can be pro-ductive only when your baby is well attached to your breast. To begin a feeding, your baby needs to be very close to you. Once attached, look at your baby's face. His or her nose and chin should be touching your breast. The broad shape of your baby's nose enables your newborn to breathe while being very close to you.

What to listen for: Now that your baby is attached, listen for rhythmic breathing. When your baby is in an active feeding pattern, you will hear the continuous rhythm of your baby's nasal breathing. Next, listen for swallows. Between breaths, your baby will ingest your milk. Your baby may gulp in quick succession when your milk is flowing fast or may briefly detach from your breast. The sounds of rhythmic breathing and swallowing are what I refer to as your baby's positive feeding signals.

What you feel: Notice what you feel during the time that you and your baby are breastfeeding. As you position your baby for a feeding, you will likely feel a grabbing sensation as your baby attaches to you. In the initial days after birth, the attachment may be somewhat painful. Some transient soreness can be normal. Once your baby has settled into a phase of productive feeding, you will feel a continuous tugging sensation. It is normal for your baby to pause and take short breaks between bursts of sucking and swallowing. As you feed your baby on one side, notice if you leak milk from the opposite breast. Leaking is a signal that your breastfeeding hormones have become activated. During this phase of milk letdown, your baby will need to swallow very quickly in an effort to keep up with the fast flow of your milk.

Record wet and dirty diapers

Although each baby is unique, healthy babies have some qualities in common. Learning how to assess your baby's overall well-being can reassure you that breastfeeding is going smoothly. Your baby's diaper count can help you in assessing overall health. If your baby is breastfeeding productively, then he or she should have multiple wet and dirty diapers daily. Wet diapers indicate that your baby is well hydrated. In the early days after birth, it may be difficult to tell if a diaper is wet, and it is normal to find pink crystal-like stains in your newborn's diaper. Following the arrival of your mature milk, your baby's diapers should be undeniably wet. Several of these diapers should feel heavy with urine.

In the early weeks of life, your breast milk has a laxative effect on your baby's intestines.[3] At least one diaper each day should be full of yellow stool and a mess to clean up! Your baby's stool might be liquid in consistency and require several baby wipes for clean-up. In addition to this large stool, your baby will have smaller bowel movements each day. Frequent stooling indicates that your baby is getting a good quantity of your breast milk. During the early weeks of life, these wet and dirty diapers tell you that your baby is productively feeding. As your baby matures, it is normal for your baby to pass stools less frequently.

Recognize feeding clusters

Besides exhibiting positive feeding signals while breastfeeding and requiring lots of diapers, a healthy baby will be eager to breastfeed. Your baby should awaken from sleep full of energy and ready to breastfeed. In addition to feedings that have a defined beginning and ending, breastfed babies will cluster feed. During a cluster or hyper-feed, your baby will actively return to the breast many times over the period of a few hours for closely linked feedings. Typically, this pattern occurs during the late afternoon or evening hours, a time of day that is challenging to mothers. Keep in mind that cluster feeding is really power feeding. By repeatedly returning to your breast, your baby is receiving small amounts of high-quality breast milk.[4] This feeding activity also serves to build your milk supply. Power feeding is a self-limiting phenomenon that your baby will eventually outgrow.

Sometimes mothers misinterpret their baby's desire to power feed as afternoon fussiness, or a mother may mistakenly believe that her breasts have run out of milk. If you are unsure about how to interpret your baby's signals, I recommend that you offer to breastfeed your baby. By offering to breastfeed you can never be wrong!

SUMMARY OF BREASTFEEDING ABCs

Establishing a breastfeeding relationship takes patience and perseverance. Once your baby is back to birth weight, you may notice that a natural feeding and sleeping pattern begins to emerge. Scheduled and timed feedings are based on formula-feeding rules and are not helpful when it comes to breastfeeding.

To judge the success of a feeding, become aware of your baby's feeding signals rather than the length of time that a particular feeding takes. If breastfeeding is going well, your baby will use numerous diapers. Additionally, most breastfed babies will have a distinct period of cluster or power feeding in the afternoon or evening. If you are ever unsure about how to interpret your baby's signals, you can never be wrong by offering a feeding.

A. ADJUSTMENT

It is normal to feel overwhelmed after you arrive home from the hospital with your newborn. It takes time for you and your baby to become adjusted to each other. Initially, it may seem that your baby needs to breastfeed in random fashion with no discernable pattern. It is easy to become frustrated with breastfeeding during this chaotic time. After this period of adjustment, you will begin to recognize your baby's natural daily patterns of hunger and sleep. This pattern won't become recognizable if you attempt to impose an artificial schedule over your baby's innate rhythm of feeding and sleeping. Remember, this rhythm won't become evident until your mature milk has arrived and your baby is back to birth weight. To ensure that your baby reaches his or her birth weight by two weeks of age, encourage your baby to feed frequently in the days after birth.

B. BECOME AWARE

Instead of watching the minutes tick by while breastfeeding, become aware of what's happening during the feeding. Observe your baby's position. Make sure your baby's nose and chin are touching your breast. Once your baby is attached, listen for the sound of your baby's rhythmic nasal breathing interspersed with swallows or gulps. These sounds are positive signals that your baby is productively breastfeeding. During a productive feeding, you should feel a tugging sensation. It is normal to feel your baby pause between active bursts of feeding. Sometimes, your baby may feed for a matter of minutes while other feedings may take longer.

C. COMPATIBILITY

Build a breastfeeding relationship with your baby that is compatible with your lifestyle. Timed feedings and rigid schedules are not conducive to breastfeeding. As a mother, you can influence your baby's overall pattern of feeding and sleeping. If it is convenient for you to breastfeed at a certain time each day, then consistently offer your baby a feeding at that time. Your baby will most likely become accustomed to this feeding. Take advantage of your body's natural rhythm and breastfeed when your breasts feel full of milk. It is normal for your baby to have a pattern of frequent or cluster feedings in the afternoon or evening. These feedings not only stimulate your milk supply but also provide your baby with small amounts of high-quality milk. By recognizing and responding to your baby's hunger and feeding signals as well as taking your own needs into account, you and your baby will develop a unique pattern of compatibility.

CHAPTER EIGHT

Getting Comfortable: How to Fit Together Perfectly for Feeding

"There must be an easier way to
hold my baby while breastfeeding."
—Deidre

When Deidre sat down to breastfeed her son Trajin, she surrounded herself with a fortress of pillows and precariously balanced Trajin on a Boppy pillow across her lap. Next, Deidre rolled herself forward, and with her arms at an impossible angle, she tried to hold her breast for Trajin. Deidre hoped he would finish breastfeeding before she got a muscle spasm in the back of her neck. When I arrived at Deidre's home for a consultation, she told me positioning was her biggest breastfeeding problem.

As soon as I saw the sofa where Deidre usually breastfed Trajin, I could guess what the problem was. The sofa was covered with an impressive assortment of breastfeeding props such as bed pillows, throw pillows, and an overstuffed, crescent-shaped Boppy pillow. Deidre found breastfeeding uncomfortable because she overused these props. Placing all of these pillows around her and under her baby distorted Deidre's natural posture. Like many mothers, Deidre caused herself further discomfort by attempting to hold her breast for Trajin throughout the entire feeding. We got started by placing Deidre and Trajin in the skin-to-skin position, and I assured Deidre that she did not need to be a contortionist to breastfeed her baby.

Deidre looked relaxed holding Trajin against her skin, and with some simple maneuvering, she could be just as comfortable while breastfeeding. Trajin had turned his head to the right, and I helped Deidre follow her son's feeding signal by assisting Trajin toward Deidre's right breast. To make it easier for Trajin to attach, I asked Deidre to press her upper arm in close to her right breast and move her right forearm under Trajin's body. This subtle maneuver shapes a mother's breast, making it easier for a baby to attach.

Deidre had been positioning Trajin straight across her lap. Instead, I suggested she try placing his body at an upward angle toward her right breast. This way, Trajin ended up right where he needed to be and easily attached to her right breast. Rather than pressing on his head, I showed Deidre how to give Trajin support with the "V" of her left hand at the level of his ears. Finally, I placed a single pillow beneath Deidre's arm so that her left wrist would not tire during feeding.

Together, we listened to Trajin's rhythmic breathing and swallowing. As the feeding progressed, Trajin adjusted his attachment and moved deeper onto his mother's breast. With his head and shoulders at an upward angle, he could keep up with the fast flow of Deidre's milk. Deidre was finally comfortable. She was able to take a deep breath and enjoy breastfeeding for the first time.

SHOULD I USE A PILLOW DESIGNED FOR BREASTFEEDING?

Positioning difficulties are usually the result of a misuse of breastfeeding props like store-bought pillows designed to wrap around a mother's waist while breastfeeding. In my experience, these pillows tend to distort a mother's natural posture while breastfeeding. A mother tends to focus on positioning the bulky pillow "just right" around her waist instead of focusing on positioning her baby at her breast. Rather than laying a young baby straight across a pillow on her lap, I teach mothers to breastfeed their infants with the baby's head and shoulders at an upward angle. Crescent-shaped lap pillows make this diagonal position impossible. My rule is simple: baby first, pillow second. As Deidre discovered, breastfeeding is much more comfortable when a mother moves her baby into position before a pillow or prop. Twins are an exception to the above statement, and positioning advice for them is offered in a later section of this chapter.

SHOULD I HOLD MY BREAST?

Besides using too many pillows, part of the reason Deidre was uncomfortable was that she held her breast like a bottle throughout every feeding. It is not necessary for a mother to hold her breast while breastfeeding. In fact, this popular practice hinders proper milk flow and can lead to plugged milk ducts. Plugged milk ducts are a painful problem that is discussed in Chapter Eleven.

If you assist your baby at the beginning of a feeding by holding your breast, gently let go of your breast after your baby becomes attached and you feel the tugging sensation of active feeding. Many mothers tell me that they habitually hold their breast out of concern over their baby's ability to breathe while breastfeeding. Your baby's face is designed for breastfeeding. The broad shape of your baby's nose enables him or her to breathe while positioned very close to your breast.

HOW DO I POSITION MY BABY AROUND MY LARGE BREASTS?

Since high school, Crystal had been self-conscious about the size of her breasts. Her breasts were so large that she had difficulty finding tops and dresses that fit around her chest. While her friends shopped for lingerie at the mall, Crystal had to order these items from a specialty store. Over the last few years, she had developed neck and shoulder pain related to the weight of her breasts. Crystal had been considering breast reduction surgery but she put these plans on hold when she became pregnant with Hallie. Pregnancy caused Crystal's breasts to become even fuller, and now that Hallie was born, Crystal wondered if it would be possible to find a comfortable breastfeeding position.

While working with Crystal, I tucked a rolled-up cloth diaper underneath her breast to bolster her breast while feeding Hallie. This small roll helped to shape and support the weight of Crystal's breast, making it easier for Hallie to maintain her attachment while feeding. Crystal wanted a clear view of Hallie's face during feedings so that she could observe Hallie's attachment and feeding signals. Before positioning Hallie, I wrapped her in a thin blanket. Next, we moved Hallie underneath Crystal's arm so that they could face each other. By supporting the lower part of Hallie's head with her hand, Crystal could easily elevate Hallie to the level of her nipple. With the weight of Crystal's breast supported by the small roll, Hallie easily attached and settled into active feeding. Finally, I placed a pillow under Crystal's arm. Crystal was surprised that she could comfortably breastfeed Hallie and still have one hand free to answer the phone.

Crystal's story is another example of how the correct placement of select props can make breastfeeding more comfortable. Sometimes, a mother may develop very heavy pendulous breasts during primary engorgement. Since effective breastfeeding is especially important during the transient time of breast engorgement, rolling a cloth diaper and placing it underneath your breast can support the weight of your breast and help your baby properly attach. Bolstering your breast in this way shapes your breast and elevates your nipple, making it easier for you to get a clear view of your baby during a feeding.

At the end of our visit, Crystal asked if she needed to change breastfeeding positions or could she continue to breastfeed Hallie in this position for all of her feedings. I encouraged Crystal as I do all my clients to master one breastfeeding position before trying something new. As long as Crystal remained comfortable, I suggested that she continue to do what works.

WHAT IS THE UNDER-THE-ARM POSITION?

As you can see by the illustration in Illustration 2, what I prefer to call the under-the-arm position is a version of what is commonly called the *football hold*. Years ago, out of the belief that language influences our everyday behavior, I renamed the football hold when working with my clients.

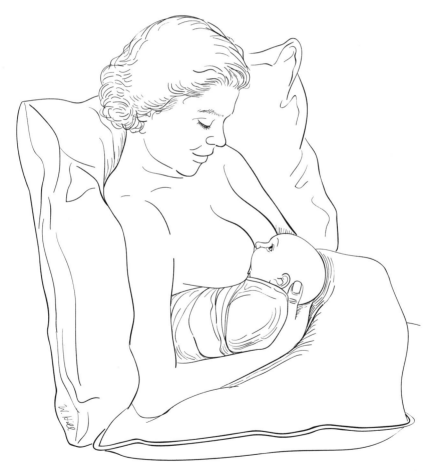

Illustration 2. Under-the-arm position

After all, a baby is not an inanimate object, and my clients lovingly hold and breastfeed their babies, not footballs. However, if sports language works for you, then by all means continue with what works!

HOW SHOULD MY NIPPLE LOOK AFTER FEEDING?

Many mothers I work with are obsessed with the appearance of their nipple after breastfeeding. Even though Barbara had a good milk supply and her son Seth was gaining weight, judging by the shape of her nipple, Barbara was convinced something was terribly wrong with the way that Seth was breastfeeding. When Seth detached, Barbara's nipple appeared squeezed from the sides instead of flattened from top to bottom like the pictures in her breastfeeding books. This concerned her enough to schedule an appointment with me, so I could take a look.

As I observed Seth breastfeeding, I noticed that Seth gulped rapidly to keep up with the flow of Barbara's milk. When he readjusted his attachment during the feeding, a surplus of milk that he could not swallow spilled from the sides of his mouth. When the feeding ended, I was not surprised to see that Barbara's nipple was laterally pinched as she had described. After seeing Seth breastfeed, I concluded that the pinched appearance was a result of Seth's effort to slow the rapid flow of his mother's milk.

Throughout the entire feeding, Barbara reported that she was completely comfortable. Since the lateral squeezing was not painful, I reassured Barbara that the shape of her nipple was not a sign of something wrong in her breastfeeding relationship. Rather, the shape of her nipple indicated that Seth could use some help to cope with Barbara's high milk supply. I suggested that Barbara hold Seth in the under-the-arm position with his head and shoulders slightly upright during feedings. Having his head elevated would help Seth to swallow and avoid feeling overwhelmed by the flow of milk at the beginning of each feeding. Naturally, the longer Seth breastfed on one breast, the flow of milk slowed and became easier for him to manage. Therefore, I suggested that Barbara encourage Seth to finish one breast before switching him to the opposite breast. Barbara easily incorporated these minor adjustments into her routine. Most important, she remained comfortable throughout each feeding, and Seth continued to thrive.

In order to receive your breast milk, your baby must be properly attached to your breast, not your nipple. During the feeding process, your baby will shape and elongate your nipple. When your baby detaches, it is normal for your nipple to appear temporarily flattened after feeding. If your nipple appears squeezed from the sides or triangular in shape, this may not be concerning unless you are experiencing pain during feeding.

HOW CAN I GET COMFORTABLE AFTER MY CESAREAN SECTION?

A cesarean section is major abdominal surgery. Getting comfortable enough to breastfeed afterward can be a challenge. If you have had a cesarean section, I recommend that you get as comfortable as possible before attempting to breastfeed so that you can focus on your baby. This may mean laying on your side to breastfeed. While on your side, there won't be any pressure on your surgical incision.

To breastfeed, simply bring your baby toward your breast that is closest to the mattress. Both of you will be lying on your sides facing each other. Make sure to start with your baby's upper lip at the level of your nipple. This should signal your baby to attach to your breast. Try putting a pillow under your head and behind your back for support so that you can relax during the feeding. If you are able to comfortably sit or recline in bed, try the under-the-arm position. This position won't put pressure on your incision, and you will be able to clearly see your baby throughout the feeding.

WHAT SHOULD I DO IF MY BABY PREFERS ONE BREAST OVER THE OTHER?

When I met Kerri, she was recovering from a difficult birth that began with an induction of labor and ended with a vacuum extraction of her daughter, Morgan. During her hospitalization, multiple nurses tried to forcibly help Kerri breastfeed Morgan by pushing and holding Morgan's head at Kerri's breast. Now that she was home from the hospital, Kerri was worried because Morgan was able to attach to only her right breast. Not only was Morgan unable to breastfeed from Kerri's left breast, but Morgan would cry hysterically when placed across Kerri's chest in preparation for feeding.

Like Morgan, most babies favor one breast over the other for breastfeeding. The fact that Morgan strongly preferred her mother's right breast may have been related to the fact that Morgan had a sore spot on her head from her birth experience. Once the soreness resolved, Kerri could easily reintroduce Morgan to feeding from the left breast. In the meantime, Morgan would get plenty of milk from the right breast, and Kerri could occasionally pump the left side and store the breast milk.

While developing a clear preference for one breast over the other can be normal, developing an aversion to the breastfeeding experience is not normal.[1] The experience of being pushed toward her mother's breast had given Morgan a negative memory of being held across her mother's chest. As feedings became more difficult, Morgan became agitated, and Kerri became frustrated. To break this negative cycle and create positive breastfeeding memories, I recommended that Kerri completely avoid upsetting Morgan during feedings. The easiest way to make breastfeeding a positive experience was to begin breastfeeding Morgan before she became too hungry and to breastfeed from a different position. To help Morgan remain calm, we wrapped her in a swaddling blanket before beginning to breastfeed. Kerri used this plan and in a matter of days, she reported that Morgan was happily breastfeeding from both breasts and seemed to have overcome her aversion.

HOW DO I GET COMFORTABLE?

Breastfeeding should be a positive and pleasurable experience for you and your baby. Position your baby for breastfeeding with confidence, not force. Never allow someone who is helping you to push your baby's head or body toward your breast. Once you and your baby find a comfortable breastfeeding position, there is nothing wrong with utilizing that same position for many days or weeks. As you view the illustrations in this book, remember that you and your baby are a unique pair designed to fit together in a unique way. These illustrations are merely meant to guide you. Feel free to customize your position as comfort dictates. Sitting on the sofa or in bed may be more comfortable than breastfeeding your baby in a narrow rocking chair or glider.

Holding your baby across your chest

Before starting, make sure you are comfortably seated on a wide chair or the sofa. Sometimes this position works best if you begin by holding your baby in the skin-to-skin position. Your baby will signal feeding readiness by turning toward one of your breasts. When this occurs, simply help your baby travel toward the chosen breast. Make sure that your nipple is near the level of your baby's upper lip; this should signal your baby to open his or her mouth up-and-over your nipple and attach to your breast. Keep your baby's head and shoulders in alignment, and avoid twisting your baby's neck. You can shape the breast that your baby is attaching to by pressing your upper arm against your side and moving the lower part of your arm beneath your baby's body. As shown in Illustration 3, your baby's head and shoulders should be angled up toward your breasts and above the level of your baby's lower body. If you need to support your baby's head, do so by forming a "V" shape with the opposite hand. You form a "V" shape with the opposite hand by spreading your thumb away from your fingers and supporting the area around your baby's ears. Listen for your baby's rhythmic breathing and swallowing. If you are holding your breast,

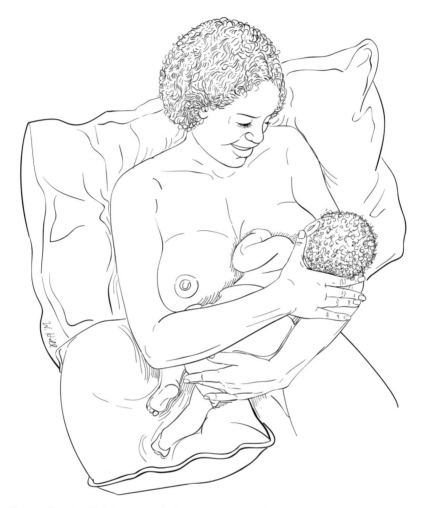

Illustration 3. Holding your baby across your chest

be sure to let go when you hear your baby's feeding signals. Finally, put a pillow under your arm to prevent your arm from tiring during the feeding.

Holding your baby under your arm

Before starting, wrap your baby in a thin stretchy blanket. This position is easier when your baby's arms and legs are contained. Next, sit comfortably and move your baby underneath your arm. Hold your baby's head with the "V" of your hand. Your baby's face should end up in front of your breast and at the level of your nipple. This should signal your baby to attach to your breast. Bring your baby in close so that your baby's nose and chin are touching your chest. If you are holding your breast, gently let go once your baby begins to actively breastfeed. Finally, put a pillow under your arm, and remember to relax your shoulders. If you have very large breasts, place a rolled-up cloth diaper underneath your breast before getting started.

Lying down with your baby

Breastfeeding while lying down, as shown in Illustration 4, may be the only comfortable position following a cesarean section or a difficult birth. Some mothers with a very high milk flow have told me breastfeeding in this position made it easier for their babies to cope with their copious milk supply. As an added bonus, this position makes nighttime feedings much easier. To start, lay down on the side that you want to breastfeed your baby. Your baby will also be on his or her side facing you. Move your baby in close so

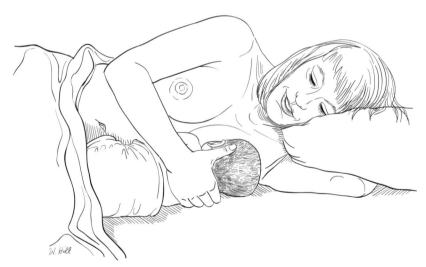

Illustration 4. Breastfeeding while lying down

that your nipple touches your baby's upper lip. Feel for your baby's attachment and active feeding. Try resting your head on your arm or a pillow.

HOW DO I POSITION MY TWINS?

After your twins are born, I recommend breastfeeding each infant separately. Feeding each baby one at a time enables you to focus on optimizing each baby's attachment before breastfeeding them together. Individualized feeding sessions also give you the opportunity to appreciate the unique characteristics of each baby. When you feel ready to breastfeed both of your babies together, I highly recommend positioning them under-the-arm style on a pillow designed for breastfeeding twins. I like the foam pillow made by Double Blessings, Inc. The angled side of the pillow helps to keep small babies in good position throughout a feeding. When your babies get bigger, you can turn the pillow over and use the level side.

SUMMARY OF BREASTFEEDING ABCs

Breastfeeding should be a comfortable experience for you and your baby. If you are uncomfortable, it may be because your body's natural posture has been distorted by too many pillows around you and underneath your baby. Many mothers make themselves uncomfortable by holding their breast while breastfeeding. It is not necessary to hold your breast. Your baby can breathe while being held close for feeding. Rather than trying to imitate a picture of someone breastfeeding, customize the position to suit your needs. For instance, if you have large breasts and want a full view of your baby's face during a feeding, position your baby's head and shoulders in front of your breast in the under-the-arm hold. Incorporate your baby's feeding style into your routine. If your baby prefers one breast over the other, begin feedings with your baby's favorite breast. Whether it's holding your baby across your chest, under your arm, or lying down, once you find a comfortable breastfeeding position, continue to use it for as long as it works.

A. ATTACH

To encourage your baby to attach deeply and comfortably to your breast, start a feeding with your nipple at the level of your baby's upper lip. Move your baby in close enough so that your baby can open up and form an attachment around or behind your nipple. Your baby's mouth doesn't need to encircle your entire areola to be properly attached. It is normal for your baby to readjust his or her mouth during a feeding.

B. BABY FIRST

When preparing to breastfeed your baby, position your baby first before adding pillows and props. Positioning your baby first preserves your natural body posture as you breastfeed. Once you feel settled, place a pillow under your arm for support. If your breasts are very heavy, you may benefit from bolstering your breast before beginning to breastfeed. To make a bolster, simply roll a cloth diaper and place it all the way underneath the breast from which your baby is going to feed. If you are breastfeeding twins together, I recommend using a pillow that is especially designed for positioning two babies.

C. CUSTOMIZE

You and your baby are designed to fit perfectly together. You will develop your own style of breastfeeding that works for the two of you. Since you are a unique pair, striving to copy exactly a picture of someone else breastfeeding her baby may not work for you. Customize the breastfeeding positions illustrated in this chapter to suit the characteristics of your body. Once you find a position that works for you and your baby, continue to use it for as long as you are comfortable.

CHAPTER NINE

How to Avoid Becoming Overwhelmed

"I came home from the hospital, and
my world was turned upside down."

—Jan

Five days after an unplanned cesarean section, Jan and baby Erika were finally home. Walking through the front door, Jan could see the house was not as she had left it. Her two attention-starved cats had used the living-room sofa as a scratching post and the ficus tree as a litter box. The answering machine was blinking urgently with five days' worth of unreturned calls. Jan decided to bypass the kitchen, and as she headed for the bedroom, Jan wondered if the pulling sensation she felt around her incision was normal. Still in her car seat, baby Erika was fast asleep. Jan couldn't remember when Erika had last been changed. With so many obligations competing for her attention, Jan didn't know what to do first after Erika was born. Exhausted and overwhelmed, Jan didn't know if she should try to get her house back in order, return phone calls, or take a nap with Erika.

After giving birth, I advise new mothers like Jan to focus on baby care, breastfeeding, and attending to their own physical and emotional well-being. These three areas offer the biggest future payoff, so they are worth the investment of your attention now. It can be difficult for a mother accustomed to a busy life outside of her home to focus inward on herself and her baby. However, having a period of time without outside obligations is valuable and will allow feelings of attachment or bonding to your baby to develop at their own pace. Of course, you can gradually expand your focus when you feel ready.

HOW DO I KNOW WHAT'S NORMAL?

The first weeks after giving birth can be a baffling time in a woman's life. Not only is your body simultaneously recovering from pregnancy and childbirth, you are also learning to anticipate the needs of your newborn. Naturally, this is a challenging time, but I have noticed that women make this time more difficult than it has to be. Too many of my clients tell me that they are overwhelmed by so many responsibilities that they hardly have time to focus on how it feels to be a new mother. They are unsure if the physical and emotional changes that they are experiencing are normal. Rather than muddling through the first weeks of motherhood trying to guess if what you are feeling is normal, I recommend learning what to expect from yourself, your baby, and breastfeeding. There is a wide range of normal experiences, and mothers recover from childbirth at their own pace, so be patient with your progress at this time.

HOW SHOULD MY INCISION FEEL AFTER A CESAREAN SECTION?

Jan had never been hospitalized before, and her cesarean section was the first surgery that she had ever had. Her time in the hospital seemed like a blur, and she was so relieved to be going home that she forgot to ask the doctor about her own recovery. Now that she was home, Jan was not sure if what she was experiencing was normal. What Jan needs to know is that a cesarean section is major abdominal surgery. As she recovers from surgery, she will have restrictions on her activity level. It is likely that she will not be able to drive a car or hold anything except baby Erika for several weeks. The pain around her incision site should gradually recede, but she might feel a pulling sensation when she moves. These sensations can be a normal part of the healing process. Jan's incision should look clean and held together. As it heals, the wound will form a scab that will fall away. The new skin underneath will look pink. Jan needs to call her doctor if she notices yellow drainage from the incision or if the incision opens up.

IS CONSTIPATION NORMAL AFTER GIVING BIRTH?

If you experienced tearing or had an episiotomy as your baby was born, that area of your body will be very sore. Any kind of movement may cause you to feel the tug and pull of your stitches. Pressure during the pushing stage of birth can cause hemorrhoids. These discomforts commonly cause a new mother to experience constipation after birth. This can also occur after a cesarean section. It takes time for your body to wake up from anesthesia, and narcotic pain relievers slow the normal movement of your intestines. This is a temporary situation. Eating high-fiber foods like bran cereal and taking an over-the-counter stool softener can help resolve postpartum constipation, so that you can concentrate on other matters!

IS BLEEDING AFTER BIRTH NORMAL?

Whether a mother gives birth vaginally or by cesarean section, she will experience a certain amount of vaginal bleeding called *lochia*. This bleeding is a normal part of having a baby. Initially, the bleeding may be like a heavy period but should lessen to a normal and then a light period as you recover. The hormone oxytocin primes your milk flow as you breastfeed your baby and also causes your uterus to contract, naturally reducing your blood loss after birth.[1] The menstrual-like cramps you feel as you breastfeed are a signal that your uterus is recovering from childbirth. Once your uterus approaches its pre-pregnancy size, this uncomfortable cramping will disappear.

WHAT IS THE DIFFERENCE BETWEEN BABY BLUES AND POSTPARTUM DEPRESSION?

During our consultation, Selena was receptive to the hands-on help that I offered as she breastfed five-day-old Bailey. An artist, Selena, had painted Bailey's nursery in magnificent swirls of blue and purple. While we sat together in Bailey's beautiful nursery, I asked Selena how she felt emotionally since becoming a mother. As Selena absorbed the question, tears filled her dark brown eyes and spilled down her cheeks. Her voice quivered as she answered, "No one has asked how I am feeling. Since having the baby, everyone asked only about Bailey." Selena went on to tell me that she was happy to finally be a mother, but that sometimes, she felt like crying for no particular reason.

Emotional lability, like what Selena described, is normal after having a baby and may be caused by shifts in a mother's hormonal landscape after birth as well as the process of adjusting to parenthood. These periods of tearfulness are often referred to as *baby blues*. Selena was relieved to know that she was not alone in her experience, and that emotional ups and downs are common after giving birth.

Baby blues or postpartum blues are very common. Nearly 85 percent of new mothers experience tearfulness and moodiness during the first week after giving birth.[2] The good news is that the blues are self-limiting, and these symptoms resolve within a few days without medical treatment. The support of family and friends can help a new mother through this challenging time.

Postpartum depression differs from the baby blues and has received a lot of media attention in recent years. Kathleen Kendall-Tackett, PhD, is an expert in the field of postpartum depression and its treatment.

Dr. Kendall-Tackett explains that unlike postpartum blues, which occur early after childbirth, a mother can develop postpartum depression anytime during the first year after having a baby. Symptoms of postpartum depression are more pronounced than the baby blues and include feelings of sadness, guilt, and despair. Symptoms can be severe and lead to thoughts of suicide. While the baby blues last a few days, symptoms of postpartum depression persist for two weeks or longer. In her book, *The Hidden Feelings of Motherhood: Coping with Stress, Depression, and Burnout*, Dr. Kendall-Tackett details the causes of depression and outlines treatment options.

Unlike the baby blues, postpartum depression may not resolve on its own. It is important that a mother seek treatment for postpartum depression not only for her own sake but for her baby's sake as well. Research has shown that a baby's emotional and social development can be affected by a mother's depression.[3] Besides talking with a qualified therapist, medical treatment may include prescription antidepressants. Many antidepressants are compatible with breastfeeding, so it is not necessary to stop breastfeeding while undergoing treatment for postpartum depression. In fact, the hormone oxytocin, released while breastfeeding, causes a mother to feel calm and relaxed, which may ease her symptoms of depression.[4] Ending a breastfeeding relationship can lead to feelings of regret and worsen a mother's depression.

This is what happened to Lorraine. She became depressed three weeks after the birth of her son Tyler. Lorraine's husband and her mother convinced her to give up breastfeeding and switch to formula. Because Lorraine was depressed, they thought that bottle-feeding Tyler would be easier on Lorraine than breastfeeding. This was not the case and Lorraine missed holding and breastfeeding Tyler. Instead of feeling better, Lorraine regretted giving up breastfeeding. She felt as if she couldn't do anything right since Tyler was born. Her depression became worse, not better. Although it is sometimes possible for a mother to recapture her lost milk supply, in the end, it is much easier to continue breastfeeding while being treated for postpartum depression.

HOW CAN I AVOID EXTRA STRESS AFTER BIRTH?

By not giving herself transition time, Georgia made the time after Carmen's birth more challenging than it had to be. Georgia and her husband, Tony, were excited to be having their first child over Thanksgiving weekend. Not wanting to disappoint any of her relatives, Georgia invited everyone to spend the holiday weekend at their house. When Georgia arrived home from the hospital with baby Carmen, she was greeted not only by her parents but by a house full of in-laws and their dogs as well. Her company settled in on the leather sofas in the living room and turned on the wide-screen television, ready for a weekend of food and football.

While Georgia retreated to the back bedroom, Carmen was held by one relative after another until she became agitated with hunger. Only then was she brought to Georgia for breastfeeding. What Georgia, her husband Tony, and baby Carmen really needed was uninterrupted time together to become acquainted and to get breastfeeding off to a successful start. Although Georgia's family thought they were being helpful by holding Carmen all day, they repeatedly missed her early hunger signals, which led Georgia and Carmen to experience breastfeeding difficulty. Georgia told me that coming home to a weekend house party was more than she could handle and that she regrets not having privacy and quiet after Carmen's birth.

To avoid unnecessary stress after birth, I recommend planning for a transition time with your baby. After coming home from the hospital, allow yourself a period of uninterrupted days or weeks without outside obligations. During this transition time, focus on yourself and your baby, not on housework or returning phone calls. Gauge how you feel. Entertaining guests is out of the question, but you may feel up for a quick visit from a coworker. During transition time, your priorities are getting to know your baby, resting your body, and breastfeeding. Spending transition time with your baby will go a long way in helping you acclimate both physically and emotionally to motherhood.

WHEN CAN I CATCH UP ON MY REST?

Jay was concerned that his wife, Simone, was lacking proper sleep because she breastfed their daughter Tess during the night. Jay was so concerned that he took matters into his own hands. One night when three-week-old Tess stirred, Jay bottle-fed her formula instead of bringing Tess to Simone for breastfeeding. By morning, Simone's breasts had become so full of milk that they were rock hard and very painful. If Jay had continued this practice of substituting bottle feedings when Tess needed to breastfeed, Simone's milk supply would have been negatively affected.

Like many new mothers, Simone found herself exhausted because she stayed awake all day and looked forward to sleeping at night. Instead of napping when Tess fell asleep during the day, Simone returned phone calls, wrote thank-you notes, or sorted the laundry. Clinging to the adult routine of being awake all day and waiting until nighttime to sleep leads to exhaustion after childbirth. Since a lack of sleep magnifies the normal emotional lability after giving birth, it is important for a new mother to take every opportunity to rest and sleep.

Instead of keeping a rigid nighttime-only sleeping pattern, I recommend that new parents temporarily shift their perspective and seize any opportunity during a twenty-four-hour period to sleep. This way, you will have more hours available for your own rest and sleep. By design, the hormones released while breastfeeding promote sleep, so take advantage of this natural phenomenon, and sleep while your baby sleeps, even if it's during the middle of the day rather than the middle of the night. Newborns are commonly awake overnight, the very hours new mothers may have counted on for sleeping. Taking a nap during the day will help you cope during the night and is preferable to having a husband or partner substitute bottle-feeding for breastfeeding.

Looking back, I wonder what I was thinking when I was a new mother. Barely a day after giving birth to my second child, Max, I put him in a sling across my chest and began vacuuming the entire house. Meanwhile, my two-year-old daughter Miriam was asleep on the sofa. This would have been an ideal time for me to take a nap. Eventually, my "I can do it all" attitude caught up with me when two weeks later, I became exhausted and called my husband in tears while he was at work.

It can be difficult to take the opportunity to rest and recover while the sink is full of dirty dishes and the baseboards need dusting. This is especially difficult for a mother who is a perfectionist. One of my clients refused all household help while recovering from a cesarean section. She wouldn't even let her mother so much as empty the dishwasher for fear of having the dishes put back out of place. Another of my clients welcomed help and temporarily hired a housekeeper to do the work that she could not while she recovered from birth. Perhaps the housekeeping approach I most admire is the simplest and came from a second-time mother who welcomed me into her easygoing living room with the warning, "I only clean up dropped or spilled food, so be careful not to trip over the books and toys on the floor."

WHAT SHOULD I KEEP TRACK OF?

Forgetfulness is common after having a baby, so it is helpful to keep simple notes to be sure that you, your baby, and breastfeeding are progressing in a positive direction. As you do this, keep in mind the information is the important part. An elaborate charting system is not necessary and will only add stress to your life. I once met a couple who devised a complex color-coded baby-care spreadsheet that covered the entire dining room table. The grids and numbers were so small that I could hardly read it. Keep the focus on your baby not on graphs and grids.

A notebook will work just fine. Use a new page each day to record the number of your baby's wet diapers and bowel movements. Also, record the number of times that your baby breastfed, if your baby woke up for the feeding, and how you felt during the feeding. Use the notebook to remind yourself to eat regularly and rest throughout the day. Again, don't wait until nighttime to sleep.

Count your baby's wet diapers

Keeping track of your baby's wet diapers is one way to gauge how well your baby is breastfeeding.[5] Wet diapers contain your baby's urine and indicate that your baby is well hydrated. After birth, expect at least one or two wet diapers each day for the first two days. If it is initially difficult to judge if your baby's diaper is wet, try putting a cotton ball in the diaper. When your baby urinates, the cotton ball will feel very wet.

As your colostrum changes to mature milk and your baby receives a greater volume of your milk, your baby will urinate more frequently. By day three or four of life, your baby's diapers should be undeniably wet. At least one diaper a day should be thoroughly soaked. Count on your baby having at least three additional damp diapers daily.

Count your baby's bowel movements

Keeping track of the number and characteristics of your baby's bowel movements is another way to gauge how well your baby is breastfeeding.[6] Your baby's first stool will be black or green in color and is called meconium. As your colostrum develops into mature milk, the color and consistency of your baby's bowel movement will change from brown and sticky to yellow and liquid.

If your baby is receiving enough breast milk, expect your baby to pass at least three stools each day by three days of age and four stools each day by four days of age. At least one of these diapers should be messy enough to necessitate changing your baby's clothes. Keep in mind that your baby's stools can vary in color; yellow, orange, even green can be normal. When your baby is requiring many diaper changes, you can be pretty sure that your baby is getting lots of breast milk. Once your baby is past his or her birth weight, it is no longer necessary to keep a written diaper count. Around four or five weeks of age, your baby's intestines mature, and it is normal for your baby to stool less frequently.

Count your baby's feedings

Your baby needs to breastfeed frequently and effectively to produce wet and dirty diapers. To be sure that your baby is getting plenty of opportunities to receive your milk, record the number of times that your baby returns to your breast over twenty-four hours. It is not helpful to time feedings. Instead notice if the feeding was productive or not. During a feeding, pay attention to your baby's position, listen for the sound of your baby's swallowing, and notice whether you feel the rhythmic tugging of active feeding. These are all signs of productive breastfeeding.

The ideal time to begin a feeding session is when your baby signals hunger. If your baby is sleepy during the first few days after birth and it is difficult for you to discern your baby's hunger signals, then gently wake your baby for feedings at least every three hours until your baby is above birth weight. Keep your baby close to you so that you can easily observe your baby's hunger signals. To ensure that your baby gets plenty of breast milk, your baby should breastfeed more than eight times in a twenty-four-hour period. In addition to feedings that have a clearly defined beginning and ending, your baby should have a period of closely linked feedings. These cluster feedings are a sign that your baby is becoming an established breastfeeder. Once your baby is regularly gaining weight, it is no longer necessary to record feedings or wake your baby to breastfeed. You can trust your baby to let you know when he or she is hungry.

DO I NEED A LACTATION CONSULTANT?

One of the reasons for counting your baby's diapers and feedings is that doing so may alert you to a problem. For instance, if a mother notices that her five-day-old baby had only passed one stool in a twenty-four-hour period, it is safe to say that her baby is not receiving enough breast milk. The problem may be that the baby is unable to attach and effectively breastfeed, or there may be a problem with this mother's milk supply. Sometimes the solution to a breastfeeding problem is as simple as ensuring that a baby feeds more frequently and from both breasts. At other times, the solution is more involved.

Many breastfeeding issues can be easily addressed by speaking over the telephone with a La Leche League leader or by attending a La Leche League meeting. However, if you feel your problem is more complex, you may require the attention of a lactation consultant. To find a certified lactation consultant, ask a La Leche League leader, your pediatrician, or the hospital to refer you to a qualified consultant. There are three basic situations that may merit an appointment with a lactation consultant.

Low diaper count

If your baby is not passing urine and stool as previously described, it may mean that your baby is not receiving enough of your breast milk. Sometimes a low diaper count indicates a problem with the development of your milk supply. Chances are if your baby is not passing urine and stool, your baby is not gaining optimal weight. A lactation consultant should help you sort through the situation and suggest specific solutions for your problem.

Pain during feeding

If you are experiencing pain when your baby breastfeeds, then, by all means, seek help. It is not normal to feel pain throughout an entire feeding or to feel pain after a feeding is over. An experienced lactation consultant should help you to identify the cause of your pain and suggest possible solutions to your problem. Potential causes of breast and nipple pain are discussed in Chapter Eleven.

Unanswered questions

As you and your baby get to know each other, your confidence in your ability to breastfeed will increase. Attending a La Leche League meeting or other breastfeeding support group may help to build your confidence. If something about the way your baby breastfeeds troubles you or if you have persistent questions about breastfeeding, then visiting a lactation consultant may put your mind at ease and increase your self-confidence in your ability to be a breastfeeding mother.

SUMMARY OF BREASTFEEDING ABCs

The first few weeks after having a baby can be a difficult time for a new mother. Not only are you recovering from pregnancy and childbirth, you are learning to care for your newborn. Setting aside a period of transition time after birth will make this time easier for you, your baby, and your family. During transition time take a break from outside obligations and spend time getting to know your baby. Take care of your own health by resting with your baby throughout the day. Don't wait until nighttime to sleep because young babies are frequently awake during the night.

Keeping track of your baby's diapers and feedings will give you an idea of how well your baby is breastfeeding. Once your baby reaches birth weight, you won't need to keep a written diaper count. Seek help if your baby has a low diaper count, breastfeeding is painful, or you have persistent questions about breastfeeding.

A. ALLOW

Allow yourself transition time after having a baby. After bringing your baby home from the hospital, plan for unstructured quiet time without outside obligations. During this time, take a break from housework and take care of yourself. Take your time getting to know your baby and let feelings of bonding to your baby develop at their own pace. You can expand your focus when you feel ready.

B. BABY BLUES

It is common after having a baby to experience baby blues or postpartum blues. Mothers may experience a period of emotional sensitivity a few days after giving birth. The baby blues will pass on its own without medical treatment. While symptoms of the blues are generally mild and short lived, symptoms of postpartum depression are more pronounced and include feelings of despair and hopelessness. A mother can develop postpartum depression any time during the first year after childbirth. Symptoms usually persist longer than two weeks and may not resolve without medical treatment. Many antidepressants are compatible with breastfeeding, so it is not necessary for a mother to end her breastfeeding relationship while being treated for postpartum depression.

C. COUNT

Keeping track of your baby's wet diapers and bowel movements can help you gauge how well your baby is breastfeeding in the initial weeks after birth. If your baby is not using enough diapers, it may indicate that your baby needs to breastfeed more frequently. Count the number of times that your baby breastfeeds in a twenty-four-hour period. Aim for more than eight feedings in twenty-four hours. In addition to frequent feedings, your baby needs to breastfeed effectively. Since timing a feeding does not indicate the effectiveness of a feeding, observe your baby's feeding signals instead of recording the passing time.

CHAPTER TEN

How to Build a Strong Supply of Mature Milk

"I want enough milk to satisfy my baby."

—Marla

recently had a home visit with Marla, who was concerned about her low milk supply. After meeting with her and her three-week-old son, Henry, I concluded that Marla's milk supply was indeed low. The cause of her trouble was clear; Henry was being cared for by a live-in baby nurse. This nurse had been keeping Henry with her during the night and for long periods during the day. Although he periodically breastfed, he was often pacified with artificial nipples and supplemented with formula bottles. Marla was young, healthy, and capable of breastfeeding. Unfortunately, frequent separation from her baby and missed breastfeeding opportunities inadvertently gave her body the message that she did not intend to breastfeed, and Marla's initially strong milk flow slowed to a mere trickle.

Your body was made to nourish your baby. During pregnancy, your breasts prepare colostrum with the assumption that you will breastfeed your newborn. After birth, this early milk gradually evolves into mature breast milk. As this occurs, the decisions that you make influence the development of your future milk supply. In the first few weeks following birth, a breastfeeding mother can take concrete steps that will lead her toward a strong milk supply. With so many variables affecting a mother's milk supply, most new mothers are unaware that many of these variables are under their control. Had Marla understood that separation, pacifiers, and bottle-feeding would have a negative impact on her milk supply, she might have decided to keep Henry with her and breastfeed him more frequently so that her milk supply could fully develop.

WHAT ARE THE SIGNS THAT MY BODY IS MAKING MILK?

Colostrum is available to satisfy your newborn's thirst and hunger immediately after birth. Small amounts of thick yellow colostrum are high in protein, minerals, and some vitamins. Interestingly, colostrum contains cholesterol.[1] Learning to metabolize cholesterol as a newborn may help your baby's body develop healthy cholesterol levels later in life. Although small in volume, these early feedings are rich in immunities that work to protect your newborn from illness. With each successive feeding, your early milk prepares your baby's stomach and intestines for the arrival of your high-volume mature milk.

Timing varies, but new mothers can expect their mature milk to "come in" three to five days after giving birth. You will know that your mature milk has arrived because your breasts will feel different, your milk will look different, and your baby will feed differently. As your early milk changes, so will your breasts. Your breasts will become bigger, heavier, and warm. Many mothers describe feeling hot or developing a transient low-grade fever when their mature milk arrives. This entire process is called *primary engorgement*.

Your newly full breasts will begin to leak, and your mature milk will have a different look from your colostrum. The color of your early milk will gradually shift from yellow to white. Compared to your early breast milk, your mature milk will be copious in volume and look watery. Even though the breast fullness of primary engorgement happens overnight, it is normal to take several days for the color of your milk to shift from bright yellow to creamy white.

Finally, you will know that your mature milk has arrived by the way your baby feeds. Compared to early breast milk, your mature breast milk is higher in volume and sweeter tasting. Like your colostrum, mature breast milk is full of living cells that work to protect your baby from illness. As your baby feeds from your newly full breast, you will hear frequent swallowing and gulping as your baby takes in larger volumes of breast milk. In response to this greater intake, your baby should have a greater output of wet diapers and bowel movements. Your baby's increasing diaper count is a sure sign of a healthy milk supply.

WHAT IS NORMAL ENGORGEMENT?

Just as the hormones of pregnancy signal your breasts to produce colostrum for your baby's first meal, the shifting hormones brought on by childbirth lead to the experience of primary engorgement. This usually occurs three to five days after birth even if a mother doesn't intend to breastfeed. How a mother contends with the onset of primary engorgement can affect her milk supply and her entire breastfeeding experience.

Tara, a second-grade teacher and new mother, handled this important phase in the development of her breastfeeding relationship just right. Tara taught up until her labor started on a Friday afternoon. Her labor quickly progressed and Carla was born early Saturday morning. Tara breastfed Carla in the delivery room and by Monday morning the new family was home. So far, Tara and Carla had sailed through their initial days as a breastfeeding couple. Suddenly, things changed. On Monday night, both of Tara's breasts became very full. It seemed that from one hour to the next, Tara's breasts grew bigger than she thought possible. Carla noticed the change and had difficulty attaching to the new shape of her mother's breast. Instinctively, Tara massaged and softened her breasts to help Carla get a better attachment. Tara breastfed Carla often, and Tara could hear Carla swallow milk as she breastfed. When Carla detached after feeding, Tara was happy to see that there was breast milk in and around her daughter's mouth.

Even with frequent feeding, Tara felt uncomfortably full. To further soften her breasts, Tara expressed a little bit of milk so that she was more comfortable. By the end of the first week following Carla's birth, Tara's breasts were full but soft. She frequently leaked breast milk and began wearing disposable nursing pads. By following her excellent intuition, Tara was able to navigate through this period of primary engorgement with her strong supply of mature breast milk intact. The uncomfortable swelling resolved and Carla was now able to easily feed from both breasts.

Tara's experience of primary engorgement was normal, or physiologic. By breastfeeding Carla frequently, Tara prevented her breasts from becoming overly distended. However, even with frequent feeding, Tara experienced the sensation of uncomfortable fullness. Overabundance at this time is normal as your body learns to predict exactly how much milk your baby needs. As Tara experienced, your body will err on the side of too much milk as opposed to not enough. As expected, within a few days, Tara's body self-regulated, and this period of engorgement passed.

Unfortunately, mishandling primary engorgement can lead a mother to experience unnecessary pain and disappointment. Because of the misinformation that Marta received when she became engorged, she ended up losing her milk supply. Marta required general anesthesia during the cesarean section birth of her son Julio. When she woke up, Julio was already in the newborn nursery. Once they got together, Marta and Julio had difficulty breastfeeding. Over the next few days, their breastfeeding troubles continued, and Julio was given formula supplements. By her fourth day in the hospital, Marta's breasts filled with milk and became very firm. However, Julio was still unable to breastfeed and therefore unable to receive Marta's milk. Throughout her hospitalization, none of the doctors or nurses recommended that Marta pump her breasts. In fact, she was told to wear a tight bra and to avoid pumping for fear of worsening her engorgement and creating more breast milk. By the time she was discharged from the hospital, nearly six days after Julio's birth, Marta's breasts were soft, and her milk seemed to be going away.

Marta really wanted to breastfeed, but Julio was unable to attach, and she didn't seem to have any milk. Once she was discharged from the hospital, Marta called and requested my help because she wasn't sure what to do next. By the time I met Marta, she had passed through her natural period of primary engorgement without ever removing any milk from her breasts. The build-up of milk coupled with the lack of regular breast stimulation caused her to lose her milk supply. Marta's body thought that she did not intend to breastfeed.

In order to preserve her milk supply and help her through the engorgement phase, hospital staff should have advised Marta to use a double electric breast pump every three hours. Not only would regular pumping serve to lessen the symptoms of painful engorgement, but Julio could have been fed his mother's pumped breast milk instead of formula. Sadly, Marta was incorrectly counseled that pumping during the early stages of engorgement would worsen her condition. This is simply not true. Early engorgement is hormonally driven, and pumping to relieve over engorgement will not worsen a mother's condition. In Marta's case, pumping would in fact have protected Marta's milk supply until Julio could learn to breastfeed. Frequent breastfeeding or pumping in the days following birth awakens receptors sensitive to the hormone prolactin, a key player in the production of mature breast milk.[2]

Marta's story has a happy ending. Marta told me she still wanted to breastfeed Julio and was eager to do whatever was necessary to recapture her lost milk supply. Marta began using an electric breast pump every few hours. She refused to be discouraged when at first her efforts produced not even a drop of milk. In the meantime, Julio continued to be supplemented with formula. Slowly, Marta's body began to respond, and she made measurable amounts of milk with each successive pumping. This motivated Marta to try a prescription medication to help restimulate her supply. Julio began breastfeeding, and, to my amazement, Marta went on to develop a very strong milk supply.

WHAT IS ABNORMAL ENGORGEMENT?

Most mothers experience the breast fullness and warmth of primary engorgement three to five days after giving birth. This is a good sign! Breast fullness harkens the arrival of your mature milk and is an indication that your body is working well. It is important to know how to navigate through this sometimes troublesome period so that you can sail smoothly into the future with your baby. Left unchecked, the normal symptoms of primary engorgement can develop into a full-blown problem.

What started out as normal engorgement for Robin quickly progressed into over engorgement. By the time Robin called me for help, she was in so much pain that she had difficulty talking. Robin's breasts were so swollen and so engorged that when I touched them during my exam, my fingers left visible indentations on her breasts. Robin explained that her milk had come in the day before and that her son Ray had been breastfeeding irregularly overnight. Robin's breasts became rock hard with no discernable nipple, making it virtually impossible for her son to attach for feeding. Robin also had a low-grade fever, a sign that her whole body was responding to the severe inflammation of her breasts.

Over the next hour, we alternated cold and heat treatments. Once the swelling abated a bit, Robin was able to pump some milk with an electric breast pump. To minimize pulling her already distended breast and nipple tissue, I instructed Robin to keep the suction on the pump low. Finally, Robin's baby was able to attach and effectively breastfeed using a nipple shield. Afterward, we once again iced Robin's breasts. Robin continued this plan until her breasts healed from the over engorgement.

Part of the reason Robin experienced such exaggerated engorgement was that Ray was her second child. Experienced mothers like Robin can expect their mature milk sooner and in greater volume than first-time mothers. Whether you are having your first baby or your fifth, it is important to know how to treat your symptoms of engorgement well before the engorgement develops into an excruciating problem.

HOW DO I TREAT MY ENGORGEMENT?

During this phase of engorgement, avoid wearing a bra. A bra may compress your breasts and make your swelling worse. Sometimes clients ask me about cabbage leaves as a treatment for engorgement. Certainly, there is no harm in wrapping your breasts in cabbage, but I prefer the treatment described next. Whatever treatment you choose, it is important to repeat the regimen every two or three hours day and night until your engorgement abates and your milk is freely flowing. Until your engorgement is under control, avoid any preparations that could potentially increase your milk production and worsen your engorgement, such as herbal teas or supplements that contain the herb fenugreek.

Cold treatment

If your breasts feel very hard and full, chances are it's not just trapped milk volume that is causing the swelling. During engorgement, your breast tissue becomes over distended and painful just like a sprained wrist or ankle. It is important to reduce the swelling so that milk flow can resume. The treatment for the breast swelling of early engorgement mimics the treatment for a sprained ankle. Before doing anything else, my treatment of choice is cold treatment. When working with an engorged mother, I insist on real ice in quart-size plastic bags. The ice can be cubed or crushed. I then wrap the bags in a thin receiving blanket and cover the mother's swollen breasts with the wrapped ice bags. I don't recommend putting ice directly against bare skin. Most mothers experience a noticeable reduction in swelling after fifteen to twenty minutes. Of course, the ice bags can be placed back in the freezer and reused. The cold treatment will need to be repeated until the engorgement is resolved.

Heat treatment

Sometimes a heat treatment is necessary to loosen a tight full breast. A heat treatment works best by getting into the shower and allowing warm water to soak the breast. The shower should be warm enough so that steam rises. Be careful not to burn your sensitive breast or nipple tissue. If you find heat helpful, then try wetting the inside of a disposable diaper with warm water and wrapping one around each swollen breast. Remove the diapers when the heat dissipates. Repeat the heat treatments frequently until your breast milk is freely flowing, and your engorgement is resolved.

Milk removal

Milk can be removed from your engorged breasts after the swelling is reduced by cold or heat treatments. Frequent milk removal is key to the healthy resolution of engorgement. Breastfeeding your baby often will help prevent your breasts from becoming over engorged. For this reason, it is important to keep your baby close to you, so you can easily breastfeed. Avoid substituting formula supplements in place of breastfeeding. Supplementing will reduce the number of times your baby breastfeeds and worsen your engorgement.

Engorgement can significantly change the shape of your breast and nipple, making it difficult for your baby to breastfeed. This can occur even when your baby has successfully breastfed prior to the development of primary engorgement. If you find yourself in this situation, then a nipple shield may help your baby reattach and effectively breastfeed. You can stop using the nipple shield once your engorgement resolves. If you are unable to breastfeed your baby, use a double electric hospital-grade breast pump every few hours. Pumping will protect your milk supply as it lessens your engorgement. Save all of your milk to feed your baby.

HOW DO I BUILD A STRONG MILK SUPPLY?

Brenda wanted to see me for a prenatal consultation because she was worried that she might not develop a strong milk supply for the baby she was expecting. Brenda was having an excellent pregnancy. Early on, Brenda's breasts felt sore, her nipples darkened, and her breasts became noticeably larger in size. Brenda was healthy and had never had breast surgery or any other risk factors that could predispose her to a low milk supply. After talking with Brenda, I assured her that the breast changes she described meant that her breasts were ready to make plenty of breast milk for her baby. After our appointment, Brenda was able to trust her body. Once her son Finn was born, Brenda followed some simple steps designed to send her body the message that she intended to breastfeed. Sure enough, Brenda developed plenty of breast milk right on schedule.

Chances are that you will build a strong milk supply to nourish your baby. Your body is well suited for motherhood, and as your milk supply matures, your body will err on the side of abundance. As I explained to Brenda, there is no shortcut to developing a strong milk supply. By putting forth effort during your baby's first few weeks of life, you and your baby can enjoy a strong milk supply later. The steps described next are designed to help you develop a full supply of mature breast milk.

Breastfeed at birth

Breastfeed as soon as possible after birth. These early feeding experiences give you a head start on your way to developing a full milk supply. Breastfeeding in the delivery room or the recovery room after a cesarean section gives your baby your early breast milk and lays the hormonal groundwork for your future supply of mature milk. Keeping your baby close to you makes getting an early start easier.

Breastfeed frequently

Breastfeed your new baby as frequently as possible. Frequent breastfeeding sensitizes your hormonal receptors to prolactin, the hormone that helps build your milk supply.[3] Once your baby is born, pregnancy hormone levels decline, and prolactin levels rise.[4] This is a crucial time in the development of your future milk supply. Breastfeeding your baby during this hormonal shift enables you to capture the crest of this prolactin wave. If you become separated from your baby or your baby is unable to breastfeed, then pump your breasts with an electric breast pump every three hours. Pumping will send your body the message that you intend to breastfeed.

Cope with engorgement

About three to five days after giving birth, your breasts will swell with the arrival of your high-volume mature milk. This signals a turning point in your breastfeeding relationship. By now, your colostrum or early milk has prepared your baby for your mature breast milk. It is important to navigate smoothly through this period of primary engorgement. Take your bra off while you are engorged to prevent compression of your breasts. If your breasts become swollen and painful, plan to use cold or heat treatments as previously described. Softening your breasts with repeated ice or heat treatments will enable your milk to flow and allow for milk removal. Breastfeed your baby or pump to prevent milk stasis and escalating engorgement. Reducing the swelling of your breasts and removing milk will preserve your future milk supply.

IS THERE ANYTHING THAT WILL INTERFERE WITH MY MILK SUPPLY?

Because so many variables impact a mother's milk supply, the cause of a low supply is not always obvious. Sometimes the origin of a mother's difficulty remains a mystery and cannot be traced back to any one cause. Of course, having a history of surgery such as breast reduction will affect a mother's potential to produce a full supply; however, she can still breastfeed,[5] as discussed in Chapter Six. Although some factors that affect milk supply are outside a mother's control, many factors are within her control.

Consider Marla, whom we met at the beginning of this chapter. Most likely, she would have developed a full milk supply if she had breastfed baby Henry early and often during the first weeks of his life instead of having him under the care of a hired baby nurse. Missing out on these early feeding opportunities suppressed Marla's milk supply.

A variety of situations or conditions have the potential to delay the arrival of a mother's mature milk. Having a difficult birth or a cesarean section may delay a mother's experience of primary engorgement.[6] Diabetics may also experience delayed primary engorgement.[7] Even being a large-size woman can put a mother's milk supply at risk.[8] Experiencing greater than expected blood loss while giving birth or having a retained placenta inside the uterus after birth can lead to milk supply problems.[9] Of additional concern are hormonal birth control measures that are prescribed or administered too early in the postpartum period.[10] Birth control hormones can short-circuit a new mother's ability to establish a full milk supply.

SUMMARY OF BREASTFEEDING ABCs

Pregnancy prepares your breasts for breastfeeding. In fact, your body assumes that you will breastfeed and prepares early breast milk for your baby's first meal. After giving birth, the hormonal landscape shifts within your body and culminates with the arrival of your high-volume mature milk. It is important to navigate smoothly through this time to protect your future milk supply. Once this phase of engorgement passes, your body will be ready to learn just how much milk your new baby needs.

A. ASSUME

Assume that you will easily build a strong supply of mature milk for your baby. If you haven't already done so, create an affirmation to that effect. If you are not sure how to do this, review Chapter One. Focus on your affirmation daily. Keep a positive breastfeeding mindset, and don't be discouraged if you have a risk factor that may predispose you for a delay in the arrival of your mature milk. I have worked with many new mothers who had multiple risk factors for delayed primary engorgement. Many of these mothers welcomed the arrival of their mature breast milk right on time. Assume you will be a breastfeeding success story, and chances are you will be.

B. BREAST CHANGES

During pregnancy, your breasts will grow larger, and the color of your nipples may darken. Your breasts will prepare colostrum for your baby's first meal. This early breast milk will be available even if your baby is born earlier than expected. About three to five days following your baby's birth, your breasts undergo more changes with the arrival of your mature breast milk. Primary engorgement is a turning point in your breastfeeding relationship. Your breasts will become larger, fuller, and warmer. The color of your breast milk will gradually change from yellow to white. Finally, your baby will respond to this high volume milk by swallowing frequently during feedings, and you may notice breast milk in and around your baby's mouth after feeding.

C. COMMUNICATE

In the hours, days, and weeks that follow your baby's birth, it is important to send your body the message that you want to breastfeed your baby. By clearly communicating your intention, your body will respond by making a strong supply of breast milk. Begin by breastfeeding after birth. Keep your baby close to you so that you can breastfeed frequently. Breastfeeding after birth and breastfeeding frequently sensitizes your body to the hormones that regulate your future milk supply. Manage the swelling that can accompany primary engorgement by applying cold or heat treatments to your breasts. Reducing the swelling of your breasts will facilitate milk removal and help you to remain comfortable.

CHAPTER ELEVEN

How to Know When Pain Is a Problem

"I heard breastfeeding hurts more than labor."

—JOCELYN

Jocelyn is pregnant with her first baby and very nervous about breastfeeding. Compared with formula, she knows that her milk will provide her baby with perfect nutrition, protection from illness, and even higher intelligence.[1] However, Jocelyn is worried that breastfeeding will be painful. As a baby, Jocelyn had been briefly breastfed, and her mother repeatedly told her that breastfeeding was so painful that she switched Jocelyn to formula. A few of Jocelyn's friends and coworkers with young children echoed similar sentiments about breastfeeding. As her pregnancy progressed, Jocelyn expected breastfeeding to be more painful than birth. By the time I met Jocelyn for a prenatal consultation, she had stocked up on bottles and formula just in case breastfeeding became too painful.

Jocelyn was given the message that breastfeeding and pain go hand in hand. Sometimes mothers get the exact opposite message of the one Jocelyn received: that breastfeeding is not only pain-free but pleasurable at every moment during every feeding. Neither message is helpful to a new mother. The truth about pain, pleasure, and breastfeeding lies somewhere between these polar opposites.

SHOULD I PREPARE MY NIPPLES FOR BREASTFEEDING?

Jocelyn began preparing her nipples for breastfeeding by rubbing them with a towel after showering. One of her friends told her this would toughen her nipples for breastfeeding. So far, all it did was make her nipples sore. During our consultation, I explained to Jocelyn that the process of pregnancy perfectly prepares her breasts and nipples for breastfeeding. There is no need to take preparatory measures, and, as Jocelyn discovered, these measures caused her nipples to become sore before her baby was even born.

DOES PAIN ALWAYS SIGNAL A PROBLEM?

The truth is that breastfeeding takes some getting used to. In the beginning, adhesions inside a new mother's nipple may need to stretch, causing some soreness. The good news is that any soreness that you feel is likely to be transient in nature and will resolve all on its own. After your mature milk arrives, you may experience breast pain related to primary engorgement. Chapter Ten discusses how to manage primary engorgement so that you can pass comfortably through that stage. During this time of adjustment, you are likely to feel many new sensations. Chances are most of what you feel is normal.

For example, I had a client who described feeling a stabbing sensation with the start of each feeding. The sensation was intense but would pass, and the rest of the feeding was comfortable. We finally figured out that the uncomfortable sensation was her milk "letting down" for her baby. The phenomenon of milk letdown, known as the *milk ejection reflex*, can be painful for some mothers. As a general rule, a painful sensation is probably not a problem if the sensation is transient in nature and is not getting worse.

On the other hand, a persistent pain that is increasing in intensity signals a problem.

SHOULD I BE AWARE OF SPECIFIC PAINFUL PROBLEMS?

Tracy called her obstetrician's office one morning after waking up with a small firm sore area on the side of her left breast. Tracy explained that she was still breastfeeding her six-week-old infant. She asked what to do. The doctor was double-booked with appointments all day, so the nurse told Tracy that she probably had mastitis and that the office would call in an antibiotic prescription later that afternoon. Had Tracy been more familiar with common breastfeeding difficulties, she would have recognized that her symptoms were consistent with a plugged duct, not mastitis. Treatment for a plugged duct includes applications of moist heat, massage, and frequent breastfeeding; not antibiotics. In fact, unnecessary antibiotic use could predispose Tracy to nipple candidiasis, another painful problem.[2]

Most health-care professionals are unprepared to assess and treat even the most common breastfeeding difficulties. Misdiagnosis leads to a delay in healing, which could harm the breastfeeding relationship. Therefore, I recommend that a mother educate herself, so that armed with knowledge, she can recognize the symptoms of a variety of common breastfeeding problems and seek appropriate treatment. Four of the most common problems that mothers in my practice have encountered are plugged ducts, breast infections, nipple trauma, and nipple infections. Along with a description of the symptoms of each painful problem, I offer a treatment plan that has worked for my clients.

Plugged milk duct

In the previous example, Tracy was suffering from a plugged milk duct. A plugged duct occurs when breast milk becomes trapped in a milk duct behind a collection of hardened milk granules or thickened milk. The plug and the backup of unexpressed milk forms a firm mass that is painful to touch. Since Tracy woke up with her plugged duct, it most likely formed during the night as Tracy missed a feeding when her baby slept longer than usual. Undrained milk in the breast can lead to the formation of plugged ducts. Other causes of plugged ducts are compressing the breast against the mattress for long periods of time while sleeping, persistently holding the breast while breastfeeding, or wearing a tight bra or baby carrier for extended periods of time.[3] Unlike a full milk duct waiting to be drained by a hungry baby, a plugged duct is very firm and very sore when touched. Although painful, isolated plugged ducts are relatively easy to remedy.

■ *Treatment*   The goal is to gently dislodge the plug and allow milk behind the plug to flow freely. If you have a plugged duct, check to be sure that your bra is not constricting any spot on your breast. Use your fingers to massage the area behind the plug. Doing some breast massage while taking a warm shower may quickly dislodge the plugged duct. After a warm shower and breast massage, breastfeed your baby. Breastfeed on the affected breast first with your baby's nose toward the painful plug. If possible, massage behind the sore area as you feed your baby.

As the plug dislodges, you may see tiny white crystals or a thick white tendril come out with your breast milk. Sometimes the plug becomes stuck within the nipple pore and forms a white milk blister, or *bleb*, which may need to be peeled away from the nipple. Don't worry if the plug dislodges while your baby is breastfeeding. It is safe for your baby to ingest.

If you are frequently afflicted with plugged ducts, examine the events that preceded the formation of your plugged ducts. For instance, you may be wearing an underwire bra or you may have missed a feeding with your baby the day before the plugged duct developed. Chronically plugged ducts may indicate that you have an abundance of milk. Adjusting your milk supply may help lessen the likelihood of repeated plugs. If you are prone to plugged ducts, avoid preparations that contain the herbal supplement fenugreek, which can increase your milk supply. A mother whom

I know struggled with painful plugged ducts for months until she realized she had overstimulated her already high milk supply by drinking large quantities of tea that contained fenugreek. Once she stopped drinking the tea, her condition improved.

Breast infection

Right from the start, Needa had a difficult time breastfeeding Javier. Her nipples quickly developed open sores, making feeding Javier painful. Once her milk came in, Needa became even more uncomfortable. Her breasts remained heavy and full, even after breastfeeding. Needa suspected Javier was not effectively draining her breasts. She tried pumping with a manual pump, but that was just as painful as breastfeeding. Needa's sister gave her some over-the-counter nipple cream, and Needa began applying it to her sore nipples. When Javier was one week old, Needa suddenly developed a fever and chills, and a large section of her left breast became red, swollen, and very painful. The next day Needa went to the doctor and was diagnosed with a severe case of infective mastitis and was readmitted to the hospital for treatment with IV antibiotics.

Needa had many factors that led her to develop infective mastitis. Her troubles started soon after birth when Needa was unable to get baby Javier comfortably attached for breastfeeding. Ineffective feedings left Needa's breasts overly full and predisposed her to developing inflammation in her breasts. The open sores on Needa's nipples served as a possible point of entry for the bacteria that ultimately led to the development of her infection. Using her sister's nipple cream may have irritated Needa's already injured nipples. When Needa went to the doctor's office, a large section of her breast had become indurated. The condition of her breast along with her high fever led to the diagnosis of infective mastitis.

By the time I met Needa, she had been discharged from the hospital and was finishing a prescription of oral antibiotics at home. Although her symptoms of mastitis had resolved and her breasts had healed, Needa remained traumatized by her experience and decided to stop breastfeeding.

■ *Treatment*   Treatment for the breast infection known as mastitis involves reducing breast swelling and curing the infection. It may be possible to avert a breast infection by treating red, inflamed breasts early on with warm showers, massage, and frequent milk removal. Milk removal can be accomplished by breastfeeding or pumping. If, however, the inflammation progresses into a full-blown breast infection, prescription antibiotics taken by mouth for ten to fourteen days are necessary.[4] Severe cases of mastitis like Needa's may require IV antibiotics.

In addition to antibiotic treatment, it is important to frequently drain milk from the affected breast either by breastfeeding or pumping. If the infection is not properly cleared, the infected area could form an abscess that may require drainage by a breast surgeon. Because many antibiotics are compatible with breastfeeding, it is not necessary to stop breastfeeding while undergoing treatment for mastitis. Your baby may notice a change in the taste of your milk. This is because the inflammation inside your breast causes a temporary shift in the salt content of your milk.[5] If breastfeeding is not possible or is too painful, it will be necessary to pump with an electric breast pump every few hours. Finally, when working with a mother who has mastitis, I advise her to discontinue over-the-counter nipple preparations, and I prescribe mupirocin and nystatin instead. This helps to heal damaged nipple tissue and may prevent the upward transfer of bacteria into the breast.

Nipple trauma

In the days following her cesarean section, Chloe was on so much pain medication that she was unaware that her nipples had become traumatized from breastfeeding. Only when Chloe began breastfeeding Lilly at home did she become aware of the painful sores on both nipples. In trying to heal the sores, Chloe began wearing breast shells under her bra and applying over-the-counter nipple preparations. Chloe seemed to have plenty of milk for Lilly, but her nipples were not improving and she began to dread breastfeeding. Chloe became especially alarmed when after a feeding there was a drop of blood from her nipple on Lilly's mouth. Chloe did not want to give up on breastfeeding, but she wasn't sure how to heal her nipples.

Chloe's nipple trauma probably occurred in the hospital but was masked by the pain medication Chloe took after her cesarean section. Now Chloe's nipples were being re-injured with each feeding. Her condition was further aggravated by using store-bought nipple cream and wearing breast shells, which served to trap body heat and humidity around her nipple. To teach Lilly to attach to the area behind the sore spots on Chloe's nipples, I suggested Chloe position Lilly in the under-the-arm hold with her nipple at the level of Lilly's upper lip. That way, Chloe could be sure that Lilly attached correctly to Chloe's breast not her nipple. Until Chloe's nipples healed, this initial attachment would be painful. With Lilly properly attached, Chloe found the rest of the feeding comfortable.

To promote healing, I prescribed two ointments that Chloe applied to her nipples after breastfeeding. She stopped using over-the-counter nipple cream and stopped wearing breast shells. To Chloe's relief, this new plan worked, and her nipples quickly improved. She looked forward to breastfeeding Lilly instead of dreading it.

■ *Treatment*   If you have nipple trauma, try breastfeeding your baby in a different position. A new vantage point will give you a better view of your baby's attachment. Afterward, allow your nipples to air dry. Avoid washing your nipples with soap, and use over-the-counter nipple preparations sparingly if at all. As your nipples begin to heal, it is normal for a scab to form and peel away from your nipple.

Be sure to use the dishwasher daily to wash breast pump parts, pacifiers, and alternative feeding devices. This will help prevent the transfer of yeast and bacteria onto your nipple. Sometimes prescription ointments are necessary to speed the healing process and prevent infection. I recommend applying mupirocin ointment and nystatin ointment to both nipples after breastfeeding or pumping. It is not necessary to wash these medications off prior to breastfeeding. Be sure to wear disposable nursing pads and change them frequently during the entire course of treatment. It may take a few weeks for your nipples to heal. Continue the treatment until your nipples are completely healed and you are able to breastfeed comfortably.

Nipple infection

Nipple trauma can lead to the development of a nipple infection.[6] This is because injury disrupts the normal skin integrity of your nipple, potentially allowing bacteria or yeast that exists on your skin to gain entry into your nipple or breast. This is especially true if your skin's usual defenses are weakened by over-the-counter nipple cream or if you have recently been exposed to antibiotics. Therefore, it is important to heal nipple trauma before nipple infection can set in. Nipple infections are very painful, and undiagnosed and untreated nipple and breast infections lead many mothers to stop breastfeeding.[7]

Petra's experience with nipple candidiasis is not uncommon. Having had the experience of breastfeeding twin boys, she knew breastfeeding could be challenging, but she knew it should not be agonizing. After Sandra was born, Petra thought breastfeeding was going well, but three weeks later, her nipples had become so sore that wearing a bra was painful. Petra wasn't sure what was wrong. Her nipples appeared normal, but they frequently burned and stung. The pain was most intense during and after Sandra fed. At her six-week check-up at the obstetrician's office, the doctor told Petra that the likely cause of her nipple pain was yeast.

Candidiasis, yeast, and thrush all refer to a fungal infection typically caused by the organism *candida albicans*. Once it gains entry and invades a mother's nipples, yeast causes nipple sensitivity, burning, and stinging.[8] A mother's nipple may appear normal, or it may look injured, red, or shiny. If a mother has symptoms of nipple candidiasis and the nipple appears normal, chances are she has a history of past nipple trauma that allowed yeast and bacteria to gain entry into her nipple tissue. The infection has the potential to affect the entire breast, in which case a mother experiences shooting and radiating breast pain. The bacterial infection staphylococcus aureus also causes nipple pain and can be mistaken for candidiasis.[9] A staphylococcus infection will cause the nipple to look raw and irritated, and under closer inspection with a flashlight, an exudate or purulent drainage may be visible on the nipple. It is not uncommon for a bacterial infection to accompany nipple candidiasis.

A baby's mouth or bottom can be affected with yeast as well. Oral thrush appears as thick white patches on the gums or tongue.[10] It can also cause a diaper rash with tiny red bumps. Both a mother and baby should be examined and, if necessary, treated together to interrupt the cycle of passing yeast back and forth.

■ *Treatment*   Human skin is not sterile. Yeast and bacteria exist as part of our normal body flora. Therefore, the goal of treatment is to reduce yeast and bacteria to a manageable level and to promote nipple healing. The treatment I prescribe for my clients is mupirocin ointment and nystatin ointment applied to both nipples after breastfeeding or pumping. These topical treatments used together for several weeks are usually very effective. If candidiasis has traveled into the breast, then a daily dose of Diflucan for two or three weeks is necessary.[11] In addition, a bacterial infection inside the breast needs to be treated with oral antibiotics.

If your baby has symptoms of oral thrush or a yeast-type diaper rash, he or she needs to be treated with nystatin or Diflucan. I recommend treating your baby's mouth with oral nystatin if you are not recovering quickly. Even if you do not see white patches in your baby's mouth, your baby could be passing candidiasis back to you. I have had a few clients whose symptoms of candidiasis did not improve with topical treatment and Diflucan. These mothers did get better after applying a dilution of gentian violet to their nipples for three mornings. Gentian violet is an old over-the-counter remedy for yeast.[12] Before applying it to your nipples, be sure to dilute it to half strength, and do not apply it to open nipple sores. As the name describes, gentian violet is purple and will stain clothing. In addition to other treatments, acidophilus from a health food store may help to increase your overall resistance to yeast.

After treating many mothers with painful nipple trauma and infections, I have observed that some of my clients retain an echo of physical sensitivity long after their symptoms have improved and their nipples have healed. They are acutely aware of any sensation, whether it's routine breast fullness or a normal letdown reflex. Even in the absence of tangible breast pain, many mothers are haunted by the memory of their infection so much so that it casts a shadow over the remainder of their breastfeeding experience.

CAN MY BABY'S TONGUE-TIE CAUSE NIPPLE PAIN?

The medical term for tongue-tie is *ankyloglossia*. The worst cases of nipple trauma that I have seen firsthand as a lactation consultant have been caused by babies with a significant tongue-tie. Ankyloglossia affects breastfeeding because the short or tight membrane called a *frenulum* under a baby's tongue limits normal tongue movement. A baby with a significant tongue-tie will be unable to maintain proper attachment while breastfeeding, and the baby's tongue will repeatedly slip back onto the mother's nipple. This leads to nipple injury, pain, and poor feedings.[13]

If your baby has a tight frenulum, it will be clearly visible when your baby cries. The frenulum looks like a thin white membrane causing your baby's tongue to appear heart shaped or with a slight cleft. Besides nipple pain, nipple injury, and mastitis in a breastfeeding mother, ankyloglossia has been associated with poor weight gain and failure to thrive in babies.[14] Without correction, older children may have speech and dentition problems. For reasons I can't fathom, pediatricians are often reluctant to assess, diagnose, or even acknowledge the significant impact tongue-tie has on mothers, babies, and the entire breastfeeding relationship. This is especially baffling because releasing a tongue-tie (called frenuloplasty) is a quick, simple office procedure.

WHO CAN HELP ME WITH A PAINFUL PROBLEM?

If you are experiencing a painful problem, it is important to seek advice from a breastfeeding ally. As discussed in Chapter Two, a breastfeeding ally is a health-care professional who values and protects your breastfeeding relationship by providing breastfeeding-friendly medical advice and prescribing medications that are compatible with breastfeeding. If you are in the midst of a painful problem, a La Leche League leader may be able to suggest possible treatment options or steer you toward a lactation consultant who can help you.

A certified lactation consultant will see you and your baby together and help you to sort through the possible causes of and solutions for your painful problem. My own experience has taught me that there is no substitute for an in-person consultation. I am not ashamed to admit that I have been fooled more than once as to the nature of a breastfeeding problem over the phone. I once counseled a mother to clear a plugged duct near her nipple. The following day, I examined the mother in person only to find that what sounded like a plugged duct turned out to be an infected Montgomery tubercle requiring treatment with antibiotics.

If your problem persists, keep looking until you find someone who has experience in treating your particular issue. A mother came to see me after being treated by her doctor for what was clearly nipple candidiasis. She faithfully followed her doctor's treatment regimen, but the burning and stinging in her nipples continued. The reason her candidiasis did not improve was that her doctor prescribed oral nystatin for her nipples instead of a topical ointment. After using the appropriate preparation, she was better in a matter of days. When it comes to breastfeeding your baby and caring for your body, be an advocate for yourself. Keep looking. There is a solution to every breastfeeding problem.

SUMMARY OF BREASTFEEDING ABCs

It is not necessary to physically prepare your nipples for breastfeeding. When your baby is born, your breasts and nipples will be ready to begin breastfeeding. As you get started, you may feel some nipple soreness. The soreness that you feel is likely temporary and will pass on its own. As the process of breastfeeding unfolds, you may feel many different sensations in your breasts and nipples. Chances are what you are feeling is normal. Not every pain signals a problem. If you feel a painful sensation and it quickly passes or resolves, it does not signal a problem in your breastfeeding relationship. On the other hand, if you experience persistent pain of increasing intensity, you may need to seek medical help for your problem. Become familiar with common breastfeeding problems so that you can advocate for appropriate treatment. You can resolve some breastfeeding problems, like a plugged duct, on your own. Other problems, such as a nipple or breast infection, may require prescription medications.

A. ANKYLOGLOSSIA

The medical term for tongue-tie is ankyloglossia. Babies born with a tight or short membrane (called the frenulum) underneath their tongue will have difficulty breastfeeding. This is because the tight or short frenulum limits the movement of the tongue. When attempting to attach to the breast for feeding, the tongue will repeatedly be pulled back and cause severe soreness and trauma to the nipple. If your baby has a tongue-tie, the thin white frenulum will be visible under your baby's tongue when your baby cries. You may notice that your baby has a heart shaped tongue or that the tongue has a cleft. The procedure to release a tight frenulum is called a frenuloplasty and is done in a doctor's office. You can breastfeed immediately following the procedure.

B. BREAST INFECTION

Signs and symptoms of the breast infection known as mastitis are a high fever, chills, and the presence of a hard red swollen area on the breast. If your breasts become inflamed, it may be possible to avert a breast infection by taking warm showers, massaging your breasts, and draining milk from your breasts. Treatment for a breast infection includes a full course of prescription antibiotics and frequent milk removal. Milk removal can be done by breastfeeding your baby or pumping with an electric breast pump. It is not necessary to stop breastfeeding while being treated for mastitis. The presence of open sores on your nipples can allow bacteria to enter the breast, so it is important to quickly heal injured nipples.

C. CANDIDIASIS

Candidiasis, yeast, or thrush refers to a fungal infection that can affect a mother's nipple and sometimes the breast. In addition to nipple sensitivity, yeast causes a burning and stinging sensation during and after breastfeeding. Yeast may cause the nipple to look irritated, or a mother's nipple may appear normal even though she may feel great pain. If the nipple appears normal, it is likely that the mother experienced nipple injury in the past that allowed yeast to enter the nipple. I treat nipple candidiasis with both mupirocin ointment and nystatin ointment applied to the nipples after breastfeeding or pumping. Sometimes a two- or three-week course of oral Diflucan is also needed to cure a yeast infection. Babies can get oral thrush or a yeast-type diaper rash. Mothers and babies should be examined and if necessary treated together to avoid reinfecting each other with candidiasis.

Phase III

*Continuing to Breastfeed Comfortably
into the Future*

After giving birth to your baby and navigating through those all-consuming first weeks of motherhood, you may feel ready to look toward the future. As you do this, you are likely to have questions about how to move forward with your baby as a breastfeeding couple. The following four chapters address the concerns that my clients have expressed as they continue to breastfeed their growing babies. As time goes on, your body naturally acclimates to breastfeeding, and you may wonder if it is normal to notice variations in the flow of your milk supply. Perhaps you have questions about venturing out and breastfeeding in public. Like most of my clients, you may wonder about the foods that you eat and if your diet is compatible with breastfeeding. Included in this phase is a chapter addressing the all-important question of how to maximize your sleep while continuing to breastfeed your baby.

CHAPTER TWELVE

How to Maintain a Strong Supply of Milk

"Sometimes I feel like I am running out of milk."

—NANCY

Nancy lives just a few blocks from the Connecticut shoreline. Her favorite pastime is to walk along the beach. When the tide is low and the water recedes, Nancy walks along the smooth new sand looking for shells. During high tide when there is more water and less beach, Nancy loves to watch the busy waves roll over each other. Last spring, Nancy and her husband, Stan, welcomed Abbie into their beach-loving family. Now safely tucked in a baby carrier, four-month-old Abbie is Nancy's constant companion on her daily walks. As a breastfeeding mother, Nancy has more in common with the tides of the ocean than she may realize.

Like the tides of the ocean she loves, Nancy's full supply of breast milk has its own daily rhythm. Instead of the gravitational pull of the distant moon, the daily tide of Nancy's milk is dictated by the complex interplay of her maternal hormones as well as Abbie's appetite. Nancy's most abundant milk flow or high tide occurs in the early and mid-morning hours. This high flow gives way to a lesser quantity of high-quality milk in the afternoon and evening hours when Abbie typically cluster feeds.

Prior to having a child of her own, Nancy worked in a daycare center. Most of the babies at the daycare center were bottle-fed on a schedule. Before feeding time, Nancy carefully measured and mixed the appropriate amount of formula for each bottle. She then held the bottle for the baby she was feeding until it was drained and empty. With bottle-feeding, each feeding was predictable.

Breastfeeding Abbie was different. Rather than a static series of feedings, Abbie's pattern varied throughout the day. Abbie seemed satisfied feeding from one breast in the morning. As the day wore on, Abbie took both breasts at each feeding. While many of the parents from the daycare center reported that their babies slept all night, Abbie needed to breastfeed once or twice during the night.

DOES BREAST MILK CONTINUALLY CHANGE?

Nancy's observations are correct. There is a tidal variation to a full milk supply. Normally, the overall volume of breast milk is greater in the morning hours and less in the late afternoon.[1] Breastfeeding from a less full breast in the afternoon provides a baby with the opportunity to access high-fat milk known as hind milk.[2] Furthermore, it is normal for one breast to make more milk than the other.[3] If a mother is unaware of these normal variations in the volume of her milk supply, she may think that she doesn't have enough milk and may unnecessarily supplement her baby with formula.

In addition to satisfying hunger, each feeding provides a baby with the optimal amount of fluid for hydration, protein for growth, and calories for energy. Unlike infant formula, all of the vitamins and minerals in breast milk are in a form that your baby can easily absorb. This means that even seemingly minute levels of vitamins and minerals in mother's milk are bioavailable, or able to be efficiently utilized by your baby. This is why breastfed babies may have less frequent stools as they mature; they literally absorb more of their mother's milk.

I use the term *responsive relationship* to describe the heartfelt interplay between a mother, her baby, and the elastic nature of a mature milk supply. Initially, the dramatic hormonal shift that occurs after a mother gives birth leads to the experience of primary engorgement. Afterward, a mother's actions or inactions play a significant role in the future development of her milk supply. Once you have cultivated a full milk supply, your breastfeeding relationship enters a dynamic new phase. Your supply of breast milk is constantly renewed, and the lactating breast is never completely empty. However, the amount of milk that a mother's breast is capable of storing varies from mother to mother and breast to breast.[4]

Your baby participates in this process by breastfeeding. By removing milk, your baby is able to clearly communicate exactly how much milk he or she needs throughout the day and during the night. Over time, you and your baby develop a unique pattern of synchronicity. Your milk volume will automatically adjust to suit the individual needs of your infant. In the event that your baby requires more milk, such as during a period of illness, the elastic quality of your milk supply will cause your supply to accommodate the needs of your sick baby. A natural benefit of the breastfeeding relationship is that it provides plenty of close physical contact during which time you and your baby communicate in mysterious unseen ways. Being together allows your immune system to recognize and respond to pathogens or germs in and around your baby's environment. Upon encountering a foreign bacteria, a mother almost immediately provides her baby with protective antibodies in her fresh breast milk.[5] From day to day and feeding to feeding, breast milk is continually updated with a fresh supply of living cells. Far from a sterile factory, a mother's breast actively responds to her environment by designing milk to meet her baby's unique needs.

SHOULD I FEED MY BABY FORMULA IN CASE MY SUPPLY IS LOW?

Cindy has been breastfeeding Taylor since birth. Taylor has been a good breastfeeder, and the pediatrician said Taylor's growth is right on track, but

Cindy was unsure that she had enough milk for Taylor. At nearly two months old, Taylor seemed hungrier than usual and wanted to breastfeed more often. When Taylor seemed especially fussy one evening, Cindy assumed that she had run out of milk and decided to open the box of formula samples that had come in the mail after Taylor was born. Taylor drank the formula but remained fussy afterward. Cindy quickly fell into the habit of feeding Taylor formula each afternoon and evening just in case she did not have enough breast milk.

Ironically, Cindy had plenty of milk for Taylor until she routinely began supplementing with formula. Instead of recognizing that Taylor was most likely experiencing a normal growth spurt or was simply fussy at that time of day, Cindy jumped to the conclusion that she had run out of breast milk. Taylor's history of excellent weight gain should have given Cindy confidence in her milk supply. All Cindy needed to do was breastfeed Taylor during this normal growth spurt or comfort her while she was fussy. Unfortunately, Cindy perceived her milk supply as low and went on to create that reality by substituting more and more bottles of formula for time at the breast. These missed feedings disrupted the responsive relationship of breastfeeding and suppressed Cindy's previously strong milk supply.

HOW CAN I TELL IF MY MILK SUPPLY IS TRULY LOW?

When assessing her milk supply, Cindy should have looked at the total picture before jumping to the conclusion that her supply was suddenly low. If you have been exclusively breastfeeding, reviewing your baby's growth pattern can help you to assess your milk supply. The fact that Taylor's growth had been normal could have served to reassure Cindy that breastfeeding was going well. If your baby has been feeding well and your supply is healthy, your baby's growth should follow a consistent curve. When assessing your breastfed baby's growth, it is important that your baby's weight is plotted on a growth curve that includes breastfed babies.

Growth curves published prior to the year 2000 represented the growth of predominantly formula-fed infants from one geographic area of the country. The revised Centers for Disease Control growth curves were compiled from a wide cross section of infants, including breastfed babies.[6] Of course, when evaluating your baby's overall growth pattern, your baby's birth weight, length, and gestational age need to be taken into account.

Naturally, your body adjusts to the process of making milk and breast-feeding your baby. As time passes, your breasts will leak less and feel less full than when you started your breastfeeding relationship. Your baby's body begins to utilize your milk more effectively, and your baby may make stools less frequently. If you are healthy and are not taking any medications known to suppress milk production, then rest assured that once you have cultivated a full milk supply, it will not disappear overnight.

Sometimes a mother's strong milk supply takes a downward turn due to a seemingly innocuous change in her breastfeeding routine. Mary had no problem establishing a plentiful milk supply for Andrew. When Andrew was about ten weeks old, Mary noticed her milk supply was trending downward. After speaking with Mary by phone, it became clear that her new nighttime routine was the cause of her recent reduction in milk supply. For the last two weeks, instead of breastfeeding Andrew when he became hungry overnight, Mary or her husband had been feeding Andrew a bottle of formula. Mary thought bottle-feeding Andrew at night provided a quick solution to the issue of nighttime feeding. Unfortunately, repeatedly missing these opportunities to breastfeed Andrew during the night resulted in an overall reduction in Mary's milk supply. This reduction occurred even though she resumed breastfeeding in the morning. Because young babies naturally feed during the night, by missing these key feedings, Mary's body got the message that she was no longer breastfeeding a young baby, and the overall volume of her milk suffered.

Infants and babies Andrew's age breastfeed during the night. Breastfeeding not only nourishes your baby, it maintains your milk supply at a level that is appropriate for the age and size of your individual baby. Once your baby begins to sleep for longer periods during the night, your body will follow your baby's cue and your milk supply will adjust accordingly. Until this naturally occurs, it is important to maintain your milk supply by breastfeeding your baby when your baby signals hunger, especially at night.

WHAT IS A TRUE LOW MILK SUPPLY?

It was not difficult to figure out why Mary's once strong milk supply became low; however, the cause of a mother's low milk supply is not always as obvious. Heather called me for an appointment because despite frequent feedings, her three-week-old son, Blake, was still below birth weight. Her pediatrician was concerned about Blake's slow growth, and Heather wasn't sure what to do next. When I met Heather, she had signs of a truly low milk supply. Although she had a healthy pregnancy and no history of any medical conditions that would predispose her to a low supply, on examination, Heather's breasts did not feel full of milk.

During our consultation, I used a specialized scale to help determine how much milk Heather had available for Blake and how effectively Blake was able to access his mother's supply. We weighed Blake in his diaper before feeding, and then I observed him breastfeed. To help increase the amount of milk available to Blake, I encouraged Heather to do some breast compression as her son slowed down each burst of active feeding. Next, we quickly switched Blake to the opposite breast and repeated the process until Blake ended the feeding on the original breast that he started with. Afterward, we weighed Blake on my scale and despite this excellent feeding session, Blake's intake was less than we hoped. Heather's milk supply was indeed low.

The good news about Heather and Blake's situation is that Heather had a milk supply to work with, and Blake was eager to breastfeed. Heather could choose to take deliberate steps in the hope of increasing her supply or she could choose to continue breastfeeding at her current level and supplement Blake with formula. Heather decided to take steps to maximize her milk supply. Next is a general guide outlining the principles that I employ when working with a mother like Heather who has a truly low milk supply.

WHAT STEPS CAN I TAKE TO INCREASE MY LOW MILK SUPPLY?

If you truly have a low milk supply, it may be possible to increase your milk production. Once again, be sure that your milk supply is indeed low. To help a mother gauge the nature of her milk supply issue, I observe a feeding and use a scale that is designed to capture even small amounts of milk taken during a feeding. If your baby is breastfeeding well and your baby's weight gain has been good, you probably have plenty of milk. If, on the other hand, you determine that your supply is low, remember that all the benefits of breastfeeding, like every interpersonal relationship, cannot be weighed and measured. Any milk that you provide your baby is of value. Whether you increase your milk volume or not, enjoy the time that you spend with your baby. Of course, each mother's situation is unique, so the advice outlined next needs to be tailored to suit your individual needs.

Supplementing

If your baby's weight gain has been slow as a result of your low milk supply, supplement your baby with your pumped breast milk or formula. As your baby gains weight, your baby's energy level and breastfeeding skills will improve. If possible, have a lactation consultant show you how to use a supplemental nursing system (SNS) while breastfeeding or use a dropper or cup feed. If you decide to use a bottle, choose one with a broad base, to remind your baby to keep his or her mouth wide open during feeding, and pace your baby's feeding so that your baby is not overwhelmed by the flow from the bottle. These measures will help to preserve your breastfeeding relationship as you increase your milk supply.

Breastfeeding

Continue to breastfeed as you build your supply. Effective, frequent breast-feeding can help to stimulate your milk supply. If your baby regularly needs a supplemental feeding, then provide your baby with part of the supplement prior to breastfeeding. Ending a feeding session by breastfeeding as opposed to some other feeding method creates a positive memory of breastfeeding for your baby. Make the most of each feeding by moving your baby from breast to breast during the feeding session. As your baby slows down on one side, quickly offer the opposite breast, and then repeat the process. This technique will naturally increase the volume of milk your baby receives from the feeding. Obviously, if you are supplementing with an SNS, keep your baby on one breast per feeding while using the device.

Pumping

Regularly using a hospital-grade double-electric breast pump for a period of time can help you to increase your milk supply. The action of pumping both breasts together sends your body a strong signal to increase production. For the purpose of increasing your supply, pump both breasts together every three hours for ten minutes on medium suction. Turning up the suction will only give you sore nipples, not more milk. If you are regularly breastfeeding your baby, try to pump for a few minutes afterward. Save all of your pumped milk for your baby. Pumping accomplishes two goals: not only does it help to increase your milk supply but it also enables you to supplement your baby with your own breast milk.

Galactagogue use

A galactagogue is a substance known to increase a mother's milk supply in conjunction with breastfeeding and pumping. The herbal supplement fenugreek is a popular galactagogue. The usual dose is three capsules taken with food three times a day.[7] Fenugreek is also available as a tea. Fenugreek capsules should be taken with food to avoid a low blood sugar reaction.

Fenugreek also causes a mother's urine to take on a sweet smell. The advantage of fenugreek is that it is inexpensive and readily available in health food stores. In my experience, fenugreek works best for mothers who are seeking to increase an established milk supply.

Mothers who have a very low milk supply may benefit from the Canadian medication domperidone (motilium). Originally prescribed to treat a gastrointestinal condition, as a side effect, domperidone increases a mother's milk supply.[8] At this time, domperidone is not approved by the FDA. In my opinion, this is unfortunate because domperidone has very few side effects, and I have seen it work very well for many of my clients. Although domperidone is safe and effective, the drug reglan (metoclopramide) has potentially serious side effects. Reglan, approved by the FDA, is also prescribed for gastrointestinal disorders and has the side effect of increasing a mother's milk supply.[9] Because of reglan's potential side effects of depression, fatigue, and anxiety, I don't recommend this medication to my clients. Remember, none of the previously mentioned galactagogues will work without effective breastfeeding or pumping.

IS IT POSSIBLE TO HAVE TOO MUCH BREAST MILK?

All her life, Bonnie succeeded at everything she tried her hand at. She sailed through college in three years instead of the usual four and had been a competitive swimmer since high school. Success came naturally to Bonnie, and when it came to breastfeeding, Bonnie wondered if her body worked too well! Her breasts filled with milk the day after giving birth to Carly. At the doctor's office a week later, Carly was not only back to birth weight but above it. Carly had too many wet and dirty diapers to count. From the surface, everything seemed perfect with breastfeeding, but two months later, Bonnie and Carly were miserable.

Even after Carly breastfed, Bonnie felt as though her breasts were too full. She didn't merely leak breast milk, she poured. Bonnie wasn't sure how to make breastfeeding a happy experience for Carly. During feedings,

Carly repeatedly pulled off and on her mother's breasts and frequently cried. Afterward, Carly sucked her fingers. Her diapers were explosive, and sometimes her bowel movements were green.

In the beginning, an abundant milk supply is normal, but by a month or so, most mothers naturally adjust to a comfortable supply. What Bonnie was experiencing two months after Carly's birth is consistent with a true oversupply of breast milk. Bonnie was uncomfortable because her breasts were constantly overfull. For her part, Carly was unable to settle into a satisfying feeding rhythm because of the fast flow and tremendous volume of Bonnie's breast milk. The fact that Bonnie's oversupply caused her to be unhappy was reason enough for her to work toward readjusting her milk supply.

Bonnie naturally made too much milk, but I have seen many mothers force their bodies into a mode of uncomfortable overproduction either by overusing a breast pump or timing feedings and arbitrarily switching breasts while breastfeeding. An oversupply of breast milk can predispose mothers to plugged ducts and mastitis. The fast flow of overly abundant milk can make it difficult for a baby to settle into an enjoyable feeding pattern.

Due to the sheer volume of milk, a baby may quickly gain a lot of weight but still feel unsatisfied after breastfeeding. This is because a baby may have difficulty accessing the slower flowing hind milk available at the end of a feeding. The steps outlined next can help you lessen an oversupply of milk. If after a month or so of breastfeeding, you have an uncomfortable oversupply, you can tailor this advice to suit your unique circumstances.

Breastfeeding

Start serial one-sided feedings. This means, breastfeed your baby on one breast per feeding and encourage your baby to completely finish a feeding on that breast. In an oversupply situation, this may necessitate returning your baby to the same breast for multiple feeding sessions. Usually doing two or three feedings in a row on one breast before switching to the opposite breast is sufficient. Bonnie's case was unusual. To balance her milk supply, Bonnie fed Carly from the left breast during the day and the right breast at night. Breastfeeding should become progressively more comfortable as your baby returns to the same breast for successive feedings.

Pumping

After beginning serial one-sided feedings, pay careful attention to the opposite breast. If it becomes uncomfortably full, you will need to pump or hand express some milk so that your breast is softer. Remember, it is the milk that is left behind in your breast that tells your body to reduce your overall volume of milk. If, however, both breasts are extremely full each morning, you could pump both breasts before beginning the process of serial one-sided feedings. Save all of the milk that you pump in the freezer to give your baby at a later date.

Medication

The decongestant Sudafed (pseudoephedrine) has the side effect of lowering or suppressing a mother's milk supply.[10] In cases of significant oversupply, taking Sudafed may help as part of your plan to lower your milk production. In rare situations of extreme oversupply, hormonal therapy in the form of hormonal birth control may be an option to consider.

HOW DO I MAINTAIN THE RIGHT AMOUNT OF BREAST MILK?

Once you have cultivated a full supply of breast milk, maintaining it is easy. As you and your baby grow together, your milk supply automatically adjusts without much effort on your part. The true beauty of a full supply of mature breast milk is that it is elastic in nature.[11] Your supply can easily accommodate shifts in your baby's needs or appetite. No longer a difficult endeavor, making milk and breastfeeding are now an effortless part of your life. This is the time to enjoy being a breastfeeding mother. Here are three principles to keep in mind as you maintain your milk supply.

Breastfeed when your baby is hungry

Your body will automatically maintain a healthy supply of breast milk to satisfy your baby's needs if you simply breastfeed your baby whenever your baby signals hunger. It is especially important to breastfeed at night if your baby awakens in hunger during the night. Nighttime feedings signal your body that you are breastfeeding a young baby and need to maintain a high volume of milk. Avoid habitually substituting pacifiers, bottles, or formula in place of time at the breast.

Be aware of medication

If you need medication, choose it consciously. Some medications have the potential to either increase or decrease your milk production. If you require medication, be sure it is compatible with breastfeeding. Many prescription and over-the-counter drugs are safe to take while breastfeeding. Doctor Hale's reference book, *Medications and Mothers' Milk*, has the most current information concerning medication and breastfeeding compatibility.

Pump your breast milk

Occasionally pumping your breast milk will not disrupt your overall milk production. Many of my clients want to pump so that their partner or husband can occasionally feed their baby. If you want to do this, then pumping and providing your own milk is always preferable to feeding your baby formula. After you have developed a full milk supply, pumping once a day will not disturb the harmony of your breastfeeding relationship.

SUMMARY OF BREASTFEEDING ABCs

Breastfeeding is a responsive relationship. Once you have established a full milk supply, you and your baby will develop a unique pattern of synchronicity that maintains your milk supply. Your supply will adjust to naturally accommodate the daily variances in your baby's appetite or need for breast milk. It is normal for you to have a greater volume of milk in the morning and less volume in the afternoon. If you have a low milk supply, it may be possible to increase your supply through effective breastfeeding, pumping, and possibly medication. Some mothers experience an uncomfortable overproduction of breast milk. Readjusting an overabundant milk supply involves one-sided feedings and some pumping.

A. ADJUST

Assess your milk supply before attempting to adjust your supply either up or down. If you are unsure if your milk supply is truly low, consider hiring a lactation consultant who will use a specialized scale to weigh your baby before and after breastfeeding. If your milk supply is truly low, you can take steps to maximize your overall milk production. This involves effective breastfeeding, pumping with an electric breast pump, and possibly taking a galactagogue.

Symptoms of breast milk overproduction include overly full breasts, excessive leaking, and feeding difficulty. Lowering your supply involves feeding your baby from one breast for multiple feedings in a row while being careful to avoid excessive fullness in the opposite breast.

B. BALANCE

Once you have established a full milk supply, maintaining the perfect balance of breast milk is easy. To keep your milk supply in balance, it is important to breastfeed when your baby signals hunger. Breastfeeding when your baby is hungry tells your body how much breast milk your baby needs. If your baby regularly wakes up during the night, it is especially important to breastfeed at that time. Breastfeeding at night stimulates your milk supply. To keep your supply in balance, avoid regular pacifier use, bottles, and formula. Many medications can increase or decrease your milk supply, so be aware of possible side effects before taking a drug. Occasionally pumping your milk will not disturb your overall balance of breast milk.

C. CHANGE

Breastfeeding is not a static experience. The volume and composition of breast milk changes throughout the day and during a feeding. The high flowing milk at the beginning of a feeding gives way to slower flowing hind milk toward the end of a feeding. The fats, proteins, vitamins, and minerals that make up breast milk are in a form that is easy for your baby to digest. The composition of breast milk is constantly changing to protect your baby from illness by producing active antibodies in response to germs and pathogens in your environment.

CHAPTER THIRTEEN

How Do I Do This in Public?
Traveling Together as a Breastfeeding Couple

"I want to be able to feed my baby
anywhere and at any time."

—CAROLYN

I was shopping at my favorite local market when I heard the unmistakable cry of a baby from the next aisle. I pushed my shopping cart around the corner, and I recognized the mother and the now contented baby. Carolyn and her baby, Owen, had been clients of mine. Carolyn was holding Owen in a sling, and it had taken her less than a minute to quiet Owen's hungry cries by discreetly shifting his position so that he could breastfeed. During our consultation, Carolyn had been eager to learn techniques that she could comfortably use to easily and privately breastfeed outside of her home.

Carolyn had easily adapted to carrying and breastfeeding Owen in a sling. This enabled her to take Owen anywhere she needed to go. Carolyn fully enjoyed the flexibility that breastfeeding gave her in her daily routine. Owen never had a bottle.

As breastfeeding becomes part of your life, you will both need and want to go out with your baby. None of the new mothers that I know want to be under house arrest during the length of time that they breastfeed their babies. As you know by now, breastfeeding is more than physical nutrition.

The mere act of breastfeeding comforts a baby who has become unsettled by unfamiliar surroundings. For this reason, planning an outing around your baby's usual feeding time is no guarantee that your baby won't need to breastfeed while the two of you keep an appointment or run an errand.

SHOULD I BRING A BOTTLE WITH ME?

Most of my clients are not as comfortable breastfeeding in public as Carolyn was. Nikki, a busy mother with three young daughters, reflected the concerns many mothers have with the notion of needing to breastfeed their baby somewhere other than at home. Nikki enjoyed breastfeeding her youngest daughter, Tamara, and wanted to make the most of her breastfeeding experience, especially because Nikki and her husband are not planning on having any more children.

Tamara was born in the late spring. Soon Nikki's two older daughters would finish their school programs for the summer. The girls were looking forward to typical summertime activities such as going to the local park, playground, and swim club. During our consultation, Nikki admitted that breastfeeding Tamara while simultaneously supervising her older daughters' outside activities was her greatest parenting concern. Nikki wasn't sure how the members of her swim club would react to seeing her breastfeed Tamara. Compared to preparing bottles of formula, breastfeeding was undoubtedly more convenient, but the thought of other people's disapproving glances caused Nikki great anxiety. Nikki decided that in addition to breastfeeding Tamara, she would regularly pump her breast milk and bottle-feed Tamara the pumped milk when on a summer outing. To have breast milk available for bottles, Nikki worked pumping into her busy child-care schedule.

Of course, I encouraged Nikki to do what would make her most comfortable. But I was sad that she felt she needed a bottle to contend with the disapproval she imagined encountering in public. Carrying a bottle for Tamara seemed redundant when Nikki had two breasts full of perfect milk ready whenever Tamara needed feeding. The fact that Nikki felt the need to bottle-feed her baby in public instead of breastfeeding speaks to the fact that we live in a formula and bottle-feeding culture. Bottle-feeding is perceived as the normal and socially acceptable way to nourish a baby. Both the real and imagined disapproval of others can be enough to cause a breastfeeding mother to carry a bottle when traveling outside her own home.

Some mothers need not travel outside their own home to feel the need to hide the fact that they breastfeed their baby. I have been on many house calls where my client is practically barricaded in the back bedroom of her home. It's as if complete physical and social isolation from the family unit as well as visitors is a price mothers must pay in order to breastfeed. One mother I worked with felt uncomfortable breastfeeding her newborn in front of her toddler. She eventually stopped breastfeeding because it became logistically impossible to continually separate herself from her toddler every time her newborn needed to be fed.

This social and physical withdrawal while breastfeeding is unnatural because the hormones that circulate in a mother's body as she breastfeeds are the same hormones that motivate us to seek the love and companionship of others.

AM I ALLOWED TO BREASTFEED IN PUBLIC?

Controversy over where a mother and her baby can or should breastfeed has spawned the lactivist movement. Lactivists support a mother's right to breastfeed her baby anywhere in the public domain. Nurse-ins have been organized in response to incidences where a breastfeeding mother has been made to feel unwelcome. Many of these nurse-ins have received national media coverage and have made breastfeeding a cause for national discussion.

No longer just a feeding choice or a women's health issue, breastfeeding has been cast into the political arena. Every mother needs to know that it is not illegal for her to breastfeed her baby anywhere in the United States.[1] Many states have enacted legislation that clearly recognizes breastfeeding as a mother's natural right. Such legislation protects mothers from being charged with a criminal offense such as indecent exposure.[2] Some states, such as Connecticut, recognize and protect a woman's right to continue her breastfeeding relationship if she reenters the workforce after having a baby. Such legislation enables a mother to pump breast milk on her breaks during the workday.

By enacting legislation that recognizes the importance of breastfeeding, states lend support to the Surgeon General's Healthy People 2010 goal of increasing the length of time to six months that a majority of mothers exclusively breastfeed their babies.[3] In order to meet the Surgeon General's goals as well as the American Academy of Pediatrics' recommendation of exclusive breastfeeding for six months and continued breastfeeding for at least one year, mothers must feel welcome to breastfeed their babies anytime and anywhere.

WHERE CAN I GO AND FEEL COMFORTABLE BREASTFEEDING?

After working with Margaret and her son Roger, I suggested to Margaret that she might enjoy attending a local mothers' group. This way she could meet other mothers in the area who had babies the same age as Roger. When I spoke with Margaret a week later, she told me that she felt that she didn't breastfeed Roger perfectly enough to attend the mothers' group. Margaret went on to say that she was intimidated at the thought of breastfeeding in front of more-experienced mothers. I was saddened by Margaret's comments. Margaret was depriving herself of companionship out of the fear of being judged by her peers. The fact is Margaret and Roger breastfed beautifully. While breastfeeding is a learned skill, it is not a competitive sport, and your performance is not ranked against other breastfeeding mothers. Nearly every breastfeeding mother I have met harbors nothing less than total support for other mothers.

When venturing out with your baby, start small. In the beginning, plan no more than a weight check at the pediatrician's office or one quick errand. As you recover from giving birth and feel more confident caring for your baby, consider a social activity like visiting a friend who is supportive of breastfeeding. Try attending a breastfeeding support group or other mothers' group with your baby. The key to a happy outing is to remain flexible in your plans and maintain a sense of humor.

I learned this lesson myself when my daughter Miriam was a baby. My husband and I were looking forward to eating an early dinner in a restaurant. While Miriam slept without stirring, we sat down in a booth, surveyed the menu, and ordered. By the time our dinner arrived, Miriam not only woke up but began to cry and would not be calmed. Miriam's cries caught the attention of the waiter who quickly returned to our table and packed our dinner to go. On the ride home, Miriam fell back asleep as if nothing had ever happened. The moral of the story is when on an outing with your baby, be prepared to make a speedy exit and remember that take-out food is always an option.

Some destinations naturally lend themselves to breastfeeding. For instance, you are likely to find plenty of privacy to breastfeed your baby in the dressing room of a clothing store. When dining out, sitting in a booth provides you and your baby more privacy than a table in the middle of a busy restaurant. In a booth, you can inconspicuously feed your baby as you enjoy your meal. The advantage of breastfeeding is that your milk is always available, no mixing or warming required. For this reason, you can breastfeed anywhere—with one exception: I don't recommend that anyone breastfeed or for that matter bottle-feed their baby in a public bathroom. A restroom is not a suitable place for food preparation or consumption of any kind.

WHAT SHOULD I WEAR?

A few wardrobe items will make breastfeeding on-the-go easier. It is worthwhile to invest in at least one high-quality nursing bra to wear under your clothes when you go out. The only bras that I recommend to my clients are Bravado bras. These bras are sized to fit a mother's body, easily unsnap for feedings, and won't constrict the circulation around your breasts. They look so beautiful when worn that after trying one on for size, a client of mine didn't want to change back into her own bra and had the store clerk ring up her sale with the Bravado bra on her body.

Besides a nursing bra, wearing a shirt designed for breastfeeding facilitates discreet breastfeeding. Nursing shirts have built-in snaps or flaps that allow you access to your breasts without lifting up or unbuttoning your shirt and exposing your torso. Before venturing out with your baby, practice breastfeeding at home in various clothing styles. Wearing what works for you will give you the confidence to breastfeed your baby in any environment. I have seen mothers attempt to conceal the fact that they are breastfeeding by draping a huge blanket over themselves and their baby. Hardly inconspicuous, these nursing curtains draw attention in the mother's direction.

The easiest way of all to travel with and breastfeed your baby in public is to carry your baby in a sling. Instead of carrying your baby around in a detachable car seat, leave the seat in the car and hold your baby in a sling. Being held close to your body will keep your baby calm, and your hands will be free during your errands. As you walk around a store, your baby will be comforted by the familiar sound and feel of your heartbeat. The rhythm and movement of your body is reminiscent of the way you carried your baby during pregnancy. A sling is versatile; it can be used to hold your baby in many different ways. Best of all, you can position your baby for discreet breastfeeding.

Sling carrying takes practice. After showing my clients how to position their baby, I recommend that they practice around the house and use the sling to take a walk around the neighborhood. If you are unable to master the sling, then try holding your baby in a front pack. While less versatile than a sling, front carriers keep your baby close to you and are better than constantly toting your baby around in a car seat. Of course, your baby still needs to be in an appropriate car seat while riding in the car.

WHAT IF I AM STILL NOT COMFORTABLE BREASTFEEDING IN PUBLIC?

If you feel uncomfortable breastfeeding your baby in a public place, scout out a more private spot in case your baby needs to breastfeed. Don't wait until your baby is crying to search for privacy. Knowing that you have a plan before your baby becomes hungry will make your day-to-day travels less stressful and more enjoyable for both of you. If you simply cannot or do not want to breastfeed your baby outside your home, you still have options. Pick an option that works for your situation and most supports your breastfeeding relationship.

Lessen the likelihood of needing to breastfeed

If your baby eats and sleeps at somewhat predictable intervals, you could try to arrange your outings around the time that your baby usually needs to breastfeed. The trouble with this plan is that being out in unfamiliar surroundings may cause your baby to become unsettled and need the reassurance of being breastfed. Also, some babies breastfeed in random fashion without a discernable pattern, making it difficult to schedule your appointments and errands around breastfeeding. To lessen the likelihood that your baby will need to breastfeed because of hunger, breastfeed before venturing out with your baby and keep the excursion short. If you don't want to breastfeed in public, you need to be prepared with an alternative feeding plan when you go out.

Pump your milk

If breastfeeding in public makes you uncomfortable, you can still provide your baby with your breast milk. Once you have established a full milk supply, pumping your milk is a breastfeeding-friendly option. To have breast milk available to take with you on your outings, plan to pump your milk in the morning after breastfeeding. Most mothers with a full milk supply have a surplus of milk in the early hours of the day. Otherwise, pump once or twice at odd times when you have the chance. Save the milk that you pump to feed your baby when you feel uncomfortable breastfeeding in public.

Keep in mind that feeding your baby with a bottle has some risks. If your baby regularly breastfeeds, he or she may have difficulty switching back and forth between your breasts and the bottle. Compared to breastfeeding, bottle-feeding probably won't calm your baby as effectively as breastfeeding will when your baby is upset and crying. Bottle-feeding instead of breastfeeding carries risks for you as well. Missing the opportunity to breastfeed your baby could cause your breasts to become overfull and lead to the development of painful plugged ducts or even a reduced supply of breast milk. While bottle-feeding your baby pumped breast milk is an option, it is not interchangeable with breastfeeding.

Give formula in a bottle

If you are uncomfortable breastfeeding in public and don't have pumped breast milk available for your baby, then feeding formula is your last choice. The milk that you make for your baby is always superior to manufactured formula, and giving formula is a much less desirable option than breastfeeding your baby or providing pumped milk in a bottle. In my opinion, the only appropriate reason to use formula is to augment or supplement a truly low supply of mother's milk.

If you use formula in place of your milk, be aware that not all preparations are ready to feed. Some formulas must be mixed or diluted. Using formula for its perceived convenience carries certain risks for your baby. Even one exposure to the ingredients in formula could potentially predispose your baby to developing a food allergy later on. Commercial formulas are more difficult to digest than your milk and may result in your baby becoming constipated.[4] Of additional concern is the fact that your baby may have difficulty switching back and forth from bottle-feeding to breast-feeding.

SUMMARY OF BREASTFEEDING ABCs

In addition to all the health benefits that breastfeeding provides to you and your baby, breastfeeding is convenient. Breast milk is always available for your baby. As you go through the day, you don't need to worry about running out of formula or washing bottles. However, many mothers are uncomfortable with the idea of breastfeeding their baby in public. The real or imagined disapproval of others can be intimidating to both new and experienced mothers. Although some breastfeeding mothers have been asked to stop breastfeeding their babies in certain public locations, it is not illegal to breastfeed anywhere. It is every mother's right to breastfeed, and it is possible to breastfeed discreetly. If you feel uncomfortable or you don't want to breastfeed your baby in public, you can try to plan short outings around the times that your baby usually feeds or bring your breast milk in a bottle.

A. ANYWHERE

Breastfeeding is convenient. One of the advantages of having a breastfeeding relationship is that you have the ability to feed your baby anywhere. Your breast milk is available at just the right temperature whenever your baby needs it. There is no measuring, mixing, or warming formula. Breastfeeding is not illegal anywhere in the United States, and you have the right to breastfeed your baby whenever your baby needs to be fed. Some states have enacted legislation that further clarifies a mother's right to breastfeed in public or pump her breast milk during the workday.

B. BRAS

Breastfeeding in public is easier when you know what to wear. Nursing bras and tops allow you to discreetly breastfeed your baby in public. Nursing bras enable you to release the cup of the bra for feedings without removing the entire garment. Nursing tops have hidden flaps or snaps that allow you to breastfeed your baby without unbuttoning your shirt and exposing your torso. Practice breastfeeding your baby at home in a variety of clothing styles until you find what works for you.

C. CARRY

Learn to carry your baby in a sling instead of toting your baby around in a car seat. Being held close to your body in a sling calms and comforts your baby, and your hands will be free as you shop or run errands. You can position your baby many different ways in a sling, including positions for discreet breastfeeding. Find someone to show you how to use a sling and practice around the house. If you are unable to master sling carrying, try holding your baby in a front pack. Although not as versatile as a sling, holding your baby close to you as you travel through your day is preferable to carrying your baby in a detachable car seat.

CHAPTER FOURTEEN

Can I Eat My Favorite Foods?
Dispelling Diet Myths

"I don't want to eat the wrong
things while breastfeeding."

—SARA

ara stood in front of her open refrigerator and contemplated quitting breastfeeding for the simple reason that she was hungry for her favorite foods and bored out of her mind from eating sliced turkey on plain bread and drinking bottled water. The pediatrician's office had given her a list of common foods like milk, cheese, and vegetables to exclude from her diet while breastfeeding. The nurse said that it would protect her baby's delicate system from upset. Sara found making dinner difficult. The lasagna her neighbors made was going to waste because it contained garlic and red sauce. Every type of salad was forbidden, and because of the spices, ordering out was definitely a no-no!

Sara started this restrictive diet because her daughter was fussy in the late afternoon. Even though she was gaining weight and breastfeeding well, the pediatrician was quick to blame Sara's diet for her baby's behavior. Sara felt guilty that her food preferences could be causing her daughter distress and vowed to stick as closely as possible to the bland foods allowed on the diet. Her daughter was still fussy, and, after a while, Sara couldn't help but wonder if formula would be better than breastfeeding.

173

Like Sara, Felice was struggling to find something to eat. When I met Felice, her mature milk had just come in, but her son Jonah was not breastfeeding effectively. The doctor's office told Felice to stick to a bland diet since she and Jonah were having breastfeeding problems. Felice's husband was an accomplished chef, and, up until a few days before, Felice had enjoyed fragrant and flavorful meals. Expertly prepared foods and fine wine were part of Felice's lifestyle. Since giving birth, Felice had gotten by on rice, potatoes, and plain pasta. Felice told me that she really wanted to learn to breastfeed Jonah but found the diet completely incompatible with her and her husband's lifestyle.

Because Jonah was not consistently breastfeeding, Felice and her husband were supplementing him with formula. Ironically, the formula was loaded with cows' milk protein—the very ingredient that the doctor instructed Felice to remove from her diet. Due to his breastfeeding difficulty, five-day-old Jonah had not breastfed effectively enough or consistently enough to experience his mother's milk, let alone become allergic to it as the doctor insinuated. During my consultation with Felice, we developed a strategy that resolved her and Jonah's breastfeeding difficulty. Felice went on to develop a full milk supply and stopped using formula. Happily, Jonah thrived on breast milk, and Felice once again enjoyed her husband's expertly prepared meals.

Common sense dictates that a baby like Jonah who has barely breastfed cannot be intolerant of his mother's breast milk. Yet this scenario is common. It seems that nearly every infant behavior is blamed on a food in the mother's diet being mysteriously transmitted to her baby through breast milk.

Analeis believed her milk caused her daughter Lola to have excessive gas and hiccups after feeding. On the advice of her pediatrician's office, Analeis fed her daughter a trial of formula instead of breastfeeding to see if her symptoms improved. If Lola's gas and hiccups resolved, the doctor reasoned, then Lola was probably allergic to something in her mother's milk. Meanwhile, Analeis watched her plentiful milk supply go to waste.

After nearly a week of formula, Lola was still gassy but had the added problem of constipation. Many young babies pass a lot of gas between feedings as a normal part of the digestive process. Lola's hiccups were most likely a reflex left over from fetal life and would occur less frequently as her body matured.

All of these mothers had been "fed" misinformation that put their breastfeeding relationship at risk. Almost every food imaginable is blamed for causing a breastfed baby's upset stomach. Although there is no proof that they are of any value, breastfeeding diets are still recommended by health-care professionals. I once visited a pediatrician who proudly shared with me a long list of foods he gave new mothers in his practice to avoid while breastfeeding. Topping the list of forbidden items were cucumbers. There is no proof of any kind that cucumbers cause harm to a breastfeeding baby. Vegetables like broccoli, fruits such as oranges, and legumes like black beans are completely digested by your body. These common foods add flavor and nutrients, not gas, to your breast milk. In fact, the daily variation in the flavor of breast milk may benefit your baby. Research has shown that babies prefer their mother's breast milk after she has eaten garlic.[1]

In the absence of a family history of food allergy, there is no benefit to eliminating foods from your diet. It makes even less sense to begin eliminating foods in the immediate postpartum period before your baby has had the opportunity to experience the full volume of your mature milk. It is highly unlikely that an allergy or intolerance to a particular food item would become evident during the immediate period after birth.

WHAT SHOULD I EAT TO MAKE HEALTHY MILK?

The savory smell of authentic Indian food welcomed me into Pradeepa and Bali's home. Pradeepa's mother had recently arrived from her home in southern India to hand prepare traditional meals for her daughter. The vegetarian recipes included legumes and vegetables and were highly seasoned with herbs known to increase a mother's milk supply. It is part of Pradeepa's culture to consume a highly spiced vegetarian diet. Nutrient-dense vegetables and beans are healthy choices for any mother and do not cause a breastfed baby gastric distress. When breastfeeding, Pradeepa's infant son will taste the foods that he will one day eat in solid form. Breastfeeding literally teaches a baby early on to prefer the flavor of the foods regularly eaten by his or her family. In keeping with her tradition, Pradeepa's mother expressed her love for her daughter by providing her with healthy meals as she recovered from childbirth.

Julie's mother was also concerned about her daughter's diet. A grandmother for the first time, she was particularly worried that Julie wasn't eating enough food and drinking enough cow's milk to produce an adequate supply of breast milk for her grandchild. During our consultation, I reassured both Julie and her doting mother that it is common for a new mother to have little appetite. As Julie's body adjusts to motherhood, her appetite would soon return to normal or even increase. I believe the phenomenon of appetite suppression in new mothers serves the purpose of enabling a mother to focus on her newborn without needing to leave her baby in order to look for food. This temporary lack of appetite would not harm the development of Julie's milk supply.

Until her appetite returned, I encouraged Julie to eat foods that she knew she digested well. A breastfeeding mother more effectively utilizes the foods she ingests.[2] This has enabled mothers to produce enough breast milk to sustain their infants throughout history when food has not been plentiful. In addition to the food she eats, a mother's body mobilizes fat stored during pregnancy to meet her energy needs. This is why a breastfeeding mother loses weight faster than a mother who doesn't breastfeed.[3]

Contrary to what her mother believed, it is not necessary for Julie to drink cow's milk in order for her to make breast milk for her baby. Cow's milk is produced by dairy cows and is designed for a calf. In no way does drinking the milk of any animal aid a woman in making breast milk for her human infant. The protein in milk and other dairy products can and does pass into mother's milk.[4] These proteins can cause a true allergy in some babies. Coping with a cow's milk protein allergy while breastfeeding is discussed in a later section of this chapter.

DO I HAVE TO DRINK A LOT OF WATER TO MAKE MILK?

Debbie was excited to be breastfeeding baby Asher, and so far things seemed to be going well. Debbie and her partner were college professors and prior to Debbie's pregnancy, they had researched the benefits breastfeeding would provide their baby. They learned that exclusive breastfeeding would increase Asher's physical and emotional health as well as make him more intelligent. Debbie was determined to breastfeed for at least a year and took leave from her academic position. Many of her friends as well as her nurse at the hospital told Debbie that she needed to drink large amounts of water to make enough breast milk to exclusively breastfeed Asher. Debbie worried that her milk supply would instantly suffer if she wasn't constantly drinking water.

It is true that breast milk is largely composed of water, but it is a myth that a mother must force herself to drink ridiculous amounts of water. Becoming overhydrated with water can confuse a new mother's body and reduce rather than increase her milk supply. It is highly unlikely that a healthy breastfeeding mother will become so dehydrated that her milk supply will become depleted. Breastfeeding naturally reminds a mother to drink water because the hormones released while breastfeeding stimulate thirst. Drinking enough fluids so that you are no longer thirsty will maintain hydration.

WILL DRINKING COFFEE AFFECT MY BABY?

Many mothers avoid caffeine during pregnancy. After giving birth, many of my clients look forward to enjoying a cup of coffee, tea, or caffeinated soda. Caffeine in these beverages causes adults to feel more awake and alert. Breastfeeding mothers often fear that caffeine will have the same effect on their baby. This is doubtful. Even large amounts of caffeine ingested by a breastfeeding mother have not been shown to be expressed in high concentrations of breast milk.[5]

My advice is to enjoy in moderation coffee and other beverages that contain caffeine. While breastfeeding, the goal is to normalize your diet and lifestyle as much as possible. If you enjoyed a coffee break in the past, there is no reason not to take one now that you are a breastfeeding mother.

CAN I HAVE A GLASS OF WINE?

Eda was planning an elaborate bridal shower for her younger sister. The event included an open bar and champagne toast. Eda had been breastfeeding her two-month-old daughter since birth and hadn't had so much as a sip of alcohol since becoming pregnant. She wanted to toast her sister's upcoming marriage and wasn't sure if having a glass of champagne was compatible with breastfeeding.

Alcohol does pass into breast milk, which mirrors the amount of alcohol a mother has consumed.[6] Having an occasional glass of wine while eating dinner is unlikely to harm a breastfeeding baby. On the other hand, rapidly swallowing back several alcoholic drinks on an empty stomach would most likely lead a mother to become inebriated, in which case, I don't recommend that she breastfeed her baby until she is sober. When it comes to alcohol, use common sense and moderate your intake. It is not necessary to pump and discard your milk after having an occasional drink.

ARE THERE FOODS I CAN'T EAT WHILE BREASTFEEDING?

Because of the risk that a food-borne illness such as listeria could potentially infect an unborn baby, it is recommended that pregnant women do not eat raw fish or soft cheeses, such as brie. However, when eaten by a breastfeeding mother, these foods do not pose a danger to her breastfed baby. In general, it is safe for a mother to eat anything while breastfeeding.

The Food and Drug Administration (FDA) recommends that breast-feeding mothers do not consume certain types of seafood.[7] Shark, swordfish, king mackerel, and tilefish all contain high levels of mercury that could pose a threat to breastfeeding infants and children. Furthermore, the FDA recommends breastfeeding mothers limit their total fish consumption to twelve ounces per week.[8] In general, shrimp, canned light tuna, salmon, pollock, and catfish contain lower levels of mercury and are considered the safest fish for a breastfeeding mother to eat.

HOW CAN I BE SURE MY MILK HAS ENOUGH OF WHAT MY BABY NEEDS?

Formula is advertised as being nutritionally complete, and after reading the list of vitamins and minerals on the back of a can of formula, Jackie wondered if her breast milk had enough of the essential nutrients that her baby needed. Nearly every mother is fully capable of making completely nutritious milk for her baby. It is true that when compared to breast milk, formula has higher amounts of certain essential nutrients. This fact misleads many mothers like Jackie to doubt the quality of their breast milk. Unlike formula, breast milk has the advantage of providing vitamins and minerals in a form that babies can fully absorb. Many of the highly concentrated ingredients in manufactured formula are simply excreted from a baby's body as waste. This is the case with iron, which is essential for the formation of red blood cells as well as normal growth and development. Breast milk contains less iron than commercial formula; however, breast-fed babies absorb nearly 50 percent of the iron in breast milk whereas the formula-fed baby is able to absorb only about 10 percent of available iron in formula.[9] Because of the high bioavailability of iron in breast milk and the fact that healthy term babies are born with a stored supply of iron, breastfed infants under six months old do not need routine iron supplements.[10] Unnecessary iron supplementation can lead to diarrhea and adversely affect a baby's growth.[11]

The concentration of water-soluble B complex vitamins and vitamin C in breast milk are influenced by a mother's diet. However, there is a saturation point or upper limit to the amount of vitamins that can be expressed in breast milk. Fat-soluble vitamins A, D, E, and K can be drawn from a mother's own vitamin stores, enabling a mother with a suboptimal diet to provide her baby with nutritious breast milk. Simply eating enough and eating a variety of foods guarantees that you will produce plenty of healthy breast milk to meet your baby's needs. However, strict vegetarians called vegans may need to take a vitamin B12 supplement.[12]

Although available in breast milk, vitamin D is meant to be gleaned from the environment through exposure to natural sunlight. Direct sunlight on the skin makes vitamin D available to the body. Because parents are aware of the dangers of overexposure to direct sunlight, many babies are not exposed to natural sunlight and, therefore, may not be getting enough vitamin D for healthy bone growth. Dark-skinned people living in northern climates are particularly at risk for vitamin D deficiency.[13] In the absence of regular exposure to sunlight, a vitamin D supplement may be necessary for exclusively breastfed babies. Currently, the American Academy of Pediatrics recommends that breastfed babies be supplemented with vitamin D starting at two months of age.[14]

DO I NEED TO SUPPLEMENT WITH FORMULA TO BE SURE MY BABY GETS ENOUGH VITAMINS?

Although she had a rich milk supply and Zac was a big healthy baby, Jackie still worried that her milk was somehow deficient. After reading that formula had more vitamin D than breast milk, Jackie began feeding formula to Zac everyday. Jackie thought of these formula feedings as vitamin supplements that would benefit her son. The fact that formula has a label and breast milk lacks one can lead a mother like Jackie to doubt the superiority of her breast milk.

It is not necessary to feed formula to an exclusively breastfed baby as a vitamin supplement. Routine bottle-feeding can disrupt a baby's ability to effectively breastfeed. Artificial formula disrupts a breastfed baby's intestinal and digestive chemistry. Frequently replacing breastfeeding with formula feeding can reduce a mother's milk supply. Exclusive breastfeeding for the first six months of life provides the greatest health and immunologic advantage to babies.

Because Jackie was concerned about the nutrient content of her milk, I suggested that she supplement herself instead of Zac. Jackie liked this idea and restarted her prenatal vitamins. She also began taking an over-the-counter fatty acid supplement. The fatty acids inherent in breast milk are thought to contribute to a baby's brain growth. Breast milk has always had the advantage of these fatty acids, but up until recently, formula has not. Jackie became confident in the completeness of her breast milk and stopped giving Zac the formula that he clearly didn't need.

WILL DIETING AND EXERCISING HARM MY BREAST MILK?

Many of my clients are eager to lose the weight that they gained during pregnancy so that they can fit back into their regular clothes. Breastfeeding automatically helps you to lose weight. Maintaining a full milk supply for your baby takes extra calories. To meet these needs, you body will mobilize the fat you stored during pregnancy. Over time, breastfeeding mothers tend to lose more weight than mothers who do not breastfeed.

It is important to recognize the fact that your body has gone through a lot of changes, and that your body won't morph back to its previous shape overnight. When choosing a weight-loss diet, I advise my clients to wait until their breastfeeding relationship is firmly established before focusing on intentional weight loss. Pick a diet that recognizes the needs of a breastfeeding mother and encourages you to eat a variety of foods. Losing weight slowly won't hurt your milk supply.

Light or moderately strenuous physical exercise won't harm the quality or taste of your breast milk. I recommend breastfeeding your baby prior to working out so that your breasts will be less full as you exercise. It is perfectly safe to breastfeed immediately after exercise. Although some exercise is healthy, obsessive exercise can have a negative impact on your breastfeeding relationship. I once had a client who initially began a breastfeeding relationship with her infant daughter, but her habitual routine of running, aerobics, and weight lifting soon interfered with her ability to breastfeed. The time this mother devoted to these daily physical activities coupled with the very rapid weight loss that resulted from overexercising led her to give up on breastfeeding.

CAN MY BABY BE ALLERGIC TO MY MILK?

Lara had been breastfeeding Grace for three months when she noticed a change in Grace's stools. Grace's bowel movements had been loose and yellow, but now her diapers contained mucous and streaks of red blood. Grace was otherwise healthy and behaving normally when Lara took her to the pediatrician. The pediatrician told Lara that Grace was allergic to her breast milk and recommended that she switch Grace to a hypoallergenic formula.

Lara didn't want to give up on breastfeeding, but she was devastated that her milk could be the cause of Grace's problem. Not knowing what else to do, she started Grace on the formula that the doctor recommended. Grace didn't like the taste, and Lara didn't like the way it smelled.

After seeking the advice of a specialist, Lara learned that Grace was not allergic to her breast milk. Rather, Grace was reacting to the cow's milk protein contained in dairy foods and present in Lara's breast milk. An allergy to cow's milk was the most likely cause of Grace's bloody stools. Proteins from dairy products in a mother's diet can leak into breast milk and cause allergic symptoms in some babies. The allergy is often expressed as bloody stools, eczema, and general discomfort. Since Grace was not happy with the taste of the formula, Lara was eager to begin breastfeeding again.

Lara began eliminating all dairy products from her diet. Besides obvious foods like milk, cheese, butter, and yogurt, cow's milk protein is often disguised as whey, casein, and lacto albumin. Dairy ingredients often lurk in breads, cookies, and cereals as well as many prepared convenience foods. Lara read labels and was vigilant about keeping her diet dairy-free. Lara once again began breastfeeding Grace, and with the new diet, Grace rarely passed an abnormal stool.

A food allergy is different from a *food intolerance*. An allergy is mediated by the immune system; an intolerance is not.[15] After ingesting the offending food item, the immune system immediately recognizes the food protein as foreign and sets off a cascade of reaction. Babies often react to an allergen by having an abnormal stool. The most severe allergic reactions occur instantly. Symptoms of severe allergy include swelling of the face, lips, and eyes. Anaphylaxis is life threatening and requires immediate medical treatment.

The most common foods that cause allergy are cow's milk, soy, eggs, peanuts, nuts, wheat, fish, and shellfish.[16] Skin testing administered by an allergist can identify which foods are causing the allergy. When a food allergy is diagnosed, it may not be a life sentence. Many babies outgrow a dairy allergy; unfortunately, peanut and nut allergies tends to be lifelong.[17] There is a range of allergic response. In highly allergic people, tiny amounts of the offending food can elicit the most severe reaction. Some individuals may be able to tolerate small amounts of the offending food but will react after eating larger amounts of the food.

Sometimes a food allergy does not become apparent until a breastfed baby is exposed to formula or starts eating solid foods. Brenda was shocked when her three-month-old daughter, Olivia, developed red hives and began to violently vomit after being fed a bottle of formula. Brenda had intended to stop breastfeeding when she went back to work. After discovering that Olivia had a dairy allergy, Brenda decided to continue breastfeeding and to pump her milk for Olivia while working.

HOW DO I MAINTAIN A HEALTHY DIET WHILE BREASTFEEDING?

While nursing you can eat almost any food that appeals to you. Best of all, you do not need to adopt a special diet to make healthy milk for your baby.

Avoid

There are very few foods that breastfeeding mothers routinely need to avoid. In general, you can eat whatever appeals to you. The exceptions are foods to which you are allergic. Food allergies can run in families, so be careful to avoid those foods to which you or someone in your immediate family are allergic. For example, if your toddler has a peanut allergy, then avoid foods that contain that ingredient for the length of time that you breastfeed your new baby. It is also recommended that breastfeeding mothers do not eat shark, swordfish, king mackerel, or tilefish because these fish contain high levels of environmental mercury.

Eat

Maintaining a full milk supply requires extra calories, so eat regularly. Satisfy your hunger with nutritious meals and snacks. Eating raw vegetables and fresh fruits will not cause your baby to become fussy. Drink to quench your thirst. It is not necessary or beneficial to force yourself to drink large amounts of water while breastfeeding. It is normal to suddenly feel thirsty or even experience the sensation of hunger while breastfeeding your baby.

Supplement

Your breast milk provides excellent nutrition for your baby. This is true even when your diet is less than perfectly balanced. It is not necessary nor is it recommended to routinely supplement your baby with formula. However, you can supplement yourself by continuing to take your prenatal vitamins. In lieu of adequate exposure to sunlight, it is recommended that breastfed babies be given a vitamin D supplement starting at two months of age.

SUMMARY OF BREASTFEEDING ABCs

You do not need to restrict your diet while breastfeeding. Simply eating a variety of foods will enable you to make a full supply of healthy breast milk for your baby. There are no special foods that you need to consume or avoid while breastfeeding. The foods that you eat on a daily basis add nutrients and flavor to your breast milk. In fact, babies are attracted to strong flavors such as garlic in their mother's milk. Spicy foods, fruits, and vegetables do not cause gas in babies. Eating a healthy diet while breastfeeding will help your baby accept solid food later on. You do not need to force yourself to drink large quantities of water or cow's milk to produce milk for your infant.

A. ALLERGY

Your baby cannot be allergic to your breast milk. However, some babies react to proteins in your breast milk from foods that you have eaten. Foods that can commonly cause a reaction in babies include cow's milk, soy, and peanuts. Symptoms of allergy in a breastfeeding baby are bloody stools, eczema, and general discomfort. If your baby is allergic to a particular food, it may be necessary to eliminate that food from your diet. In the case of cow's milk protein, it is important to read the labels of all the foods that you eat. Dairy ingredients are commonly added to everyday foods. The diagnosis of a food allergy may not be lifelong. Many babies outgrow their allergy.

B. BEVERAGE

Contrary to popular belief, it is not necessary to drink excessive amounts of water to make a full milk supply. Drinking enough water so that you are not thirsty will keep you adequately hydrated. A healthy mother will not suddenly become dehydrated. Mothers do not need to drink cow's milk to produce breast milk. It is a myth that drinking the milk of an animal contributes to the production of human milk. In fact, some babies have a negative reaction to the proteins in cow's milk. It is safe for a breastfeeding mother to drink coffee while breastfeeding. Occasionally drinking alcohol is unlikely to harm your breast milk or your baby.

C. CONSUME

Consume a variety of healthy foods while breastfeeding. Fruits and vegetables do not cause gas in breastfed babies because your body digests these foods. Seasoned and spicy foods add flavor to your breast milk. Babies like the varied flavor of breast milk. The concentration of certain vitamins in your breast milk varies with your diet while other vitamins can be drawn from stores in your body. Breast milk provides excellent nutrition for a baby even when a mother's diet is not optimal.

CHAPTER FIFTEEN

Yes, You Can Get Some Sleep

"Losing sleep is the hardest part of being a mom."

—Sofie

When I arrived at Sofie and Larry's house for our 9 A.M. appointment, both new parents were exhausted. Larry had dark circles beneath his eyes, and it looked as though he had not shaved in several days. As we sat down in the living room, Sofie looked equally sleep deprived. She tearfully explained that she did not think she could continue breastfeeding her one-week-old daughter because she was so exhausted.

Sofie and Larry described their newborn as having her days and nights mixed up. During the day, baby Missy would sleep for several consecutive hours between feedings, but by nightfall, she would awaken and not return to sleep for any measurable amount of time. Throughout the night, Sofie and Larry took turns trying to console Missy. When Missy seemed sleepy, they would return her to her crib in the nursery. In short order, Missy would reawaken and begin to cry.

Sofie found the logistics of nighttime feedings exhausting. Each time that Missy needed to be fed, Sofie got up from her own bed, traveled to the nursery, turned on the light, lifted Missy from her crib, and placed her on the changing table to check her diaper. Finally, the pair would sit to-gether in the glider and breastfeed. With the current state of affairs, no one in the family was getting any rest during the night. Larry and Sofie were baffled by their new baby and unsure if breastfeeding was to blame for Missy's nighttime wakefulness.

I quickly reassured Larry and Sofie that there was nothing wrong with their daughter. It is common for a young baby like Missy to have erratic waking and sleeping patterns.[1] During the first weeks of a newborn's life, the secret to sleep is not found in night-lights, glow toys, or lullabies. Nighttime wakefulness is the result of biology. In the beginning, breast-fed babies like Missy are hungrier at night than during the day. Your new-born's hunger naturally corresponds to the rise of your breastfeeding hormones after midnight.[2] These late-night feedings serve to help a new mother like Sofie build a strong milk supply. Missy is naturally drawn to her mother during the night not only for breast milk but for the sensa-tion of warmth and security as well.

Larry and Sofie were exhausted and miserable because they were working against rather than with Missy's inborn biology. My approach is to work with and around a baby's innate nighttime needs while helping parents get as many consecutive hours of sleep as possible. Over time, the situation will evolve, and your baby will sleep more at night and be awake for more hours during the day.[3]

To make the necessary adjustments to Larry's and Sofie's nighttime routine, we moved our consultation from the living room to the couple's master bedroom. Instead of getting up each and every time to breastfeed Missy in a chair, I taught Sofie how to breastfeed Missy while lying down in bed. This position encouraged Sofie to rest and take advantage of the breastfeeding hormones that naturally promote relaxation. I also advised moving Missy's seldom used bassinet to the bedside. Using the bassinet would save both parents from traipsing back and forth to the nursery. To further streamline baby care, I helped Larry set up a portable diaper changing station in their bedroom. With these simple adjustments, Sofie and Larry were able to enjoy more hours of sleep while continuing to breastfeed Missy.

SHOULD I WAKE MY BABY UP AT NIGHT?

Unlike Missy, two-week-old Marco slept without stirring for nearly six hours at night. Marco's mother, Cheryl, was delighted that her new baby was such a sound sleeper. When Cheryl wondered whether Marco should be awakened for breastfeeding during the night, her mother-in-law advised her to "never wake a sleeping baby." During my consultation with Cheryl, the reason for Marco's sound sleep became clear.

Marco was not gaining weight; in fact, he had lost several ounces since leaving the hospital. Sleeping for long periods of time was Marco's way of conserving energy. Young babies can easily fall into a pattern of sleeping for long stretches and skipping feedings. To keep this from happening, I recommend gently waking your baby up to breastfeed during the night. Holding your baby or changing your baby's diaper should be enough to arouse your sleepy baby for a feeding. Once your baby is above birth weight, it is no longer necessary to wake your baby up at night. The two of you will establish a natural pattern of feeding and sleeping during the day as well as during the night.

SHOULD I SLEEP WITH MY BABY?

A few years back, I was invited to a baby shower. As is customary, the mother-to-be opened her gifts during the party. She received fancy baby clothes, a car seat, and assorted baby toys. One gift struck me as curious. It was an ordinary looking stuffed animal that when activated by a switch on its back made the extraordinary sound of a beating heart. The stuffed animal with the fabricated heartbeat was designed to comfort a newborn in place of its human mother. Without a doubt, every baby is born with an innate longing to be held across its mother's heart. Nowhere else is a baby assured protection from cold, hunger, and loneliness. It is a mistake to believe that a baby born to seek the sound and smell of its own mother could for a single second be satisfied by the mechanical rhythm of an artificial heart.

Babies are born to be near their mothers day and night. It's human nature, pure and simple. In recent years, sleeping together or co-sleeping has been a topic of debate. The advantages of co-sleeping are obvious. Being physically close to your baby enables you to breastfeed your baby with minimal effort and enables you to get more sleep.[4] Chances are that the two of you will share similar sleep states. Being close together during the night helps your baby to naturally awaken from a deep sleep at appropriate intervals. In this way, co-sleeping and breastfeeding throughout the night help your baby to establish a healthy sleep pattern that may prevent sudden infant death syndrome (SIDS).

Critics of co-sleeping fear that a young baby could become entrapped in blankets or pillows in a parent's bed or that an adult may accidentally injure a baby while moving in their sleep. Additionally, there is the potential risk that a baby could fall out of an adult bed. The debate continues as to whether co-sleeping truly reduces the risk of SIDS.[5] Sometimes parents are not focused on safety issues but are instead concerned that their baby will have trouble transitioning to his or her own space for sleep after sleeping in the parents' bed.

Over the years, I have found that people have strong feelings about whether or not it is appropriate to sleep with their baby. I am repeatedly baffled by parents who balk at the notion of keeping their baby next to them through the night, yet these same people regularly invite the family dog to share space in their bed. Whether you take advantage of the ease that co-sleeping provides for a few nights or many months, some considerations will make sleeping together safer. Don't sleep with your baby on a water bed. Don't position your baby on the edge of your bed or sofa. Remove fancy pillows and extra bedding from your sleeping space, and don't co-sleep if either you or your partner has consumed alcohol.

Finally, consider using a co-sleeper unit that attaches to your bed; this way, your baby will have a safe space next to you and at the level of your own bed.

SHOULD I LET MY BABY CRY TO SLEEP?

Greta was planning on going back to work part-time when her daughter Shannon was four months of age. Greta had hoped that Shannon, now three months old, would be sleeping through the night before she returned to work. A friend told Greta about a foolproof training method that will get any baby to sleep all night alone in a crib. Shannon still slept in a bassinet at her parents' bedside and breastfed during the night. Greta and her husband decided to give the plan a try and were hopeful that Shannon would soon sleep in her crib all night long.

The very next night Greta bathed and breastfed Shannon and put her in the crib, dimmed the nursery lights, and left the room exactly as the training program dictated. Shannon had never been left alone in a dark room before, and she instantly sensed something was amiss. Her smile quickly faded, and she began to wail. When her parents didn't answer her call, her crying soon reached a hysterical pitch. Meanwhile, as mandated by the plan, Greta and her husband waited outside the nursery door and watched the clock for the prescribed number of minutes to pass before they were to check on little Shannon.

The plan permitted no hugging or holding. Greta was to briefly look in on Shannon and exit in no-nonsense fashion. When she finally reentered Shannon's room, Greta did not recognize the baby she saw when she peered over her daughter's crib railing. Gone were Shannon's delicate dimples, giggles, and gummy smiles. This little girl's face was wet with tears and contorted in terror. Shannon's desperate sounding cries were briefly interrupted as she gasped for air. Greta wasn't sure what to do. She had never seen Shannon so distraught, and yet the sleep-training program clearly discouraged prolonged parental contact. Pampering and coddling at this time would interfere with Shannon's ability to learn to sleep all night in her crib. As Greta pondered all of this, Shannon's face darkened, and she violently vomited.

Greta realized she had made a mistake. Leaving her daughter alone to cry in a dark room went against the grain of her mothering instinct. This method of sleep training did not fit her parenting style, which was based on unconditional love and trust. In a heartbeat, she retrieved Shannon from her crib, held her, and claimed back her trust.

Allowing a baby to cry hoping that the baby will learn to sleep can damage a mother's ability to instinctively respond to her baby. A colleague of mine shared with me a disturbing story about a mother who repeatedly left her baby to cry at night all alone in a crib. Over time, the mother built up a tolerance of sorts to the sounds of her baby's cries, so much so that she became desensitized to the most compelling cry of all: the cry of her child's pain. One particular night, the baby woke up crying and the mother remained in her own bed and ignored the crying. Over an hour had passed and the baby was still crying. Finally, the mother checked on her baby, who was burning hot with fever and in desperate pain from an ear infection.

Habitually turning a deaf ear to a baby's cries damages a mother's ability to respond to the subtle nuances of her baby's voice, and it goes without saying that being left to cry erodes the trust a baby has in his or her mother. Letting your baby cry at night breaks the physical, emotional, and hormonal connection that you have built with your baby through breastfeeding.

One of the advantages of cultivating a breastfeeding relationship with your baby is that you will intuitively read between the lines of your baby's behavior. Through your breastfeeding experience, you will develop a keen sense of your baby's needs that lasts long after your breastfeeding relationship had ended. You will know that your child is sick before the thermometer detects a fever. You will sense an impending growth spurt well before the scale registers a weight gain. You will smell fear in a dark bedroom well before your child calls out to be rescued from an imaginary nemesis in a nightmare.

SHOULD I LET MY BABY FALL ASLEEP WHILE BREASTFEEDING?

According to the National Sleep Foundation website, nearly 50 million Americans suffer from some type of sleep disorder.[6] As a testament to these statistics, multiple television commercials market prescription sleep aids directly to the consumer. Mattress companies advertise expensive bedding virtually guaranteed to lull exhausted adults to sleep. Perhaps we would have less difficulty falling asleep as adults if we had developed positive associations with falling asleep as babies. Nothing provides your baby with a stronger sensation of security than being held and breastfed before sleep. Yet many mothers are told that sleeping at the breast is a bad habit and are advised not to allow their babies to fall asleep while breastfeeding. This advice robs a baby of the opportunity to develop a pleasant association with sleep and gives rise to sleep difficulty.

Stephanie received a popular baby care book at her baby shower that recommended mothers avoid allowing their babies to fall asleep while breastfeeding. Instead of sleeping, the book counseled mothers to engage their babies in play after breastfeeding. Stephanie wanted her baby to be a good sleeper, and after her daughter Maisy was born, Stephanie did her best to follow the advice outlined in the book. The trouble was that toward the end of each feeding Maisy fell into a very deep sleep and could not be aroused for play. As Stephanie and Maisy discovered, falling asleep after becoming satiated at the breast is a physiologic response, not a matter of choice. Maisy was simply lulled to sleep by the action of breastfeeding and her mother's milk.

Breast milk contains hormones that contribute to feelings of contentment and sleepiness. These hormones relax a mother as well. Biology intended for Stephanie and Maisy to rest together following a feeding.

Engaging in any activity other than sleep after breastfeeding defies Mother Nature. Falling asleep after breastfeeding is a normal developmental stage. There will be plenty of opportunity for playful activity as your baby matures. For the time being, take advantage of the opportunity to rest and sleep with your baby. Falling asleep while breastfeeding will not cause poor sleep habits.

WILL BOTTLE-FEEDING HELP MY BABY SLEEP AT NIGHT?

Although it is impossible to force an unwilling baby to breastfeed, it is possible to force a less-than-willing baby to bottle-feed. I knew a couple who habitually bottle-fed their baby pumped breast milk every evening. The baby was sleeping just fine and drank the bottle without fully waking up. The parents believed the feeding extended the infant's sleep cycle. Chances are the extra feeding given when the baby was asleep and not hungry disturbed rather than promoted the baby's sleep cycle.

Giving your baby breast milk in a bottle won't necessarily make your baby sleep longer at night, but once you have an established breastfeeding relationship, having your husband or partner occasionally feed your baby during the night probably won't cause any harm. Keep in mind that drinking from a bottle may not satisfy your baby's need to be close to you the way breastfeeding does. However, if you want your baby to take a feeding from a bottle so that you can have a few hours of uninterrupted sleep, be sure to breastfeed or pump before going to bed. This will lessen the likelihood of developing a plugged duct. If your baby regularly wakes up hungry at night, it is important for the well-being of your milk supply to breastfeed at night. When your baby sleeps for longer stretches, your milk supply will naturally adjust.

WHEN SHOULD MY BABY SLEEP LONGER AT NIGHT?

All babies eventually stop waking up to breastfeed at night. When a baby stops waking up at night is highly individualized and dependent on a baby's overall growth, developmental stage, and daytime feeding pattern. For instance, it can be normal for a well-grown four-month-old to sleep from midnight to 5 A.M., and it can be just as normal for an eight-month-old to awaken and breastfeed during these same hours. It is also common for a baby who usually sleeps for a long stretch at night to unexpectedly awaken at night when approaching a developmental milestone like walking or speaking. Breastfeeding helps to ease your baby's passage through these life-changing transitions. As always, breastfeeding provides not only nutrition and calories but also the reassurance that makes advances in your baby's physical growth and emotional development possible. Of course, if your baby is sick, breastfeeding at night will comfort your baby; moreover, the antibodies in your breast milk are like medicine that speeds your baby's recovery.

Besides being physically tired, parents bear the additional burden of feeling that a baby who wakes up at night may be less than perfect. It's as if a baby's character is judged on nighttime sleep habits. A baby who does not need to wake up at night is judged to be a good and considerate citizen. On the other hand, a baby who requires more attention during the night is deemed as difficult, even selfish. These labels are assigned by parents, healthcare providers, or even complete strangers who have no relation to the baby in question.

I am reminded of a baby girl whom I came across while waiting in line at the post office one afternoon. I could not help but overhear a mother behind me in line discussing her baby's sleep habits with the woman waiting beside her. Although several customers separated us, the mother's voice was loud enough for me to catch wind of her words as she complained about her daughter waking up during the night. Her baby was strapped in her car seat carrier, which rested on the post office floor. As the line inched forward, the mother briefly lifted the seat by the handle and set it back down in front of her feet. The mother was telling an acquaintance that her baby did not sleep through the night because she had become spoiled and stubborn. She went on to say that she used a remote video monitor to observe her baby as she cried. Seeing nothing that could cause her daughter distress, she determined that her baby was crying without reason and did not answer her baby all night.

I shifted in line just enough to get a glimpse of the baby girl. The girl's eyes were open, but her mother, still engaged in conversation, seemed not to notice that her baby was awake. The baby girl had sparse strands of blond hair pale enough to be considered white. Her long eyelashes were the same shade of pale as the wisps of her hair. She was gazing about, but from her vantage point on the post office floor, her crystal blue eyes were incapable of catching and holding anyone's attention. The clerk summoned me forward. With my package weighed, stamped, and on its way, I lost track of the fragile-looking little girl.

I can't help but think of her and wonder if her mother answers her cries at night or if the baby has given up on crying altogether. Contrary to what you may have heard, holding and breastfeeding your baby during the night will not spoil your baby or cause your baby to become a poor sleeper. Meeting your baby's needs now will prevent your baby from becoming anxious and fearful during the night, and, in the end, your baby will become a better sleeper.

WHAT CAN I DO TO GET MORE SLEEP AT NIGHT?

The reality of having a new baby means that you will sleep less at night. This is temporary. When your baby is very young, he or she needs to breastfeed during the night. This phase will pass, and your baby will eventually sleep through the night. Working with your baby instead of against the flow of your baby's hunger will help you to maximize your sleep while meeting your baby's need to breastfeed during the night.

Sleep when you can

Seize every opportunity to rest and sleep. Instead of waiting for your traditional bedtime, take an afternoon or evening nap. Sleep later in the morning or go back to sleep after feeding your baby. Look for a natural lull in afternoon activities so that you can rest with your baby. Resting in the afternoon will give you more patience and stamina to cope during the night. Silence the ringer on your phone and cell phone so that you won't be tempted to answer calls. You will be in a better frame of mind to talk after you have gotten a bit of rest.

Breastfeed lying down

Avoid getting up when you don't have to. As discussed in Chapter Eight, practice breastfeeding your baby while lying on your side during the day so that you can comfortably do this at night. Conserve energy by minimizing the need for physical activity during the night. Keep your baby close to your bed. Consider investing in a co-sleeper unit that attaches to the side of an adult bed. Keep diapers and baby wipes nearby so that you won't need to search for these essential items in the middle of the night. Avoid turning on bright lights by using a flashlight at night.

Pump occasionally

If you want a few consecutive hours of sleep without breastfeeding your baby, you can pump your breast milk and have your partner feed your baby. If your baby is older and has been breastfeeding well, it is unlikely that this occasional practice will harm your breastfeeding relationship. When giving your baby a bottle, it is always preferable to use your own milk and not formula. While occasionally pumping and skipping a night-time feeding won't disturb the circadian rhythm of your milk production, routinely substituting bottles for breastfeeding can have a negative impact on your supply.

SUMMARY OF BREASTFEEDING ABCS

It is normal for your baby to wake up and breastfeed throughout the night. Breastfeeding at night develops and maintains your milk supply. Once your baby is regularly gaining weight, it is no longer necessary to wake your baby at night. Make things easier on yourself by keeping your baby close to you at night. Minimize the need to get up and out of bed by learning to breastfeed your baby from the side-lying position. It is natural for you and your baby to become sleepy at the end of a feeding. Take advantage of this opportunity to rest with your baby. Nighttime waking is a phase that will pass, and your baby will eventually sleep at night.

A. ACKNOWLEDGE

Acknowledge the fact that your baby will wake up during the night. In the beginning, having a baby means that you will sleep less. To help you cope with this inevitable situation, rest and sleep whenever you can during the day. Some babies seem to need more attention during the night than others. This is a temporary situation. Holding and breastfeeding your baby at night will not spoil your baby or cause your baby to become a poor sleeper. The time that you spend comforting and caring for your baby at night will pay off. Eventually, both you and your baby will sleep through the night.

B BIOLOGY

Babies are biologically driven to wake up during the night. These nighttime feedings match the natural rise of your breastfeeding hormones. Breastfeeding at night serves to build and maintain your milk supply. Your baby naturally craves the warmth and protection of being close to you. Falling asleep at the end of a feeding is normal. The action of breastfeeding as well as your breast milk cause your baby to feel sleepy. Take advantage of the fact that you and your baby were meant to rest and sleep together after a feeding. Sleeping after breastfeeding will not cause your baby to become a poor sleeper later in life.

C. CO-SLEEPING

Sleeping with your baby, or co-sleeping, makes breastfeeding virtually effortless at night. Having your baby next to you in bed can increase the amount of sleep that you and your baby are able to get at night. By sleeping together, you and your baby will automatically have similar sleep cycles. Co-sleeping and breastfeeding throughout the night naturally promotes a healthy sleep pattern. Critics of co-sleeping point out that a baby can become entrapped in adult bedding, fall out of bed, or become injured by a restless adult. To make co-sleeping safe, avoid waterbeds, remove extra pillows from your bed, and don't co-sleep if either you or your partner has consumed too much alcohol.

Phase IV

Developing Your Own Happy Ending

In order to have a happy breastfeeding relationship with your baby, breastfeeding must comfortably fit into the greater context of your family life. Phase IV addresses issues modern mothers are likely to contend with. A chapter on family life discusses how breastfeeding affects your romantic relationship and how a breastfeeding mother can incorporate romance into her life. Like many mothers, you may wonder if it is possible to continue breastfeeding your baby after rejoining the workforce. An entire chapter provides you with a strategy for protecting your milk supply as well as preserving your breastfeeding relationship in the workplace. Eventually, you and your baby will stop breastfeeding. The final two chapters explore the process of weaning as well as how to choose healthy foods for your baby that complement rather than replace breastfeeding.

CHAPTER SIXTEEN

How to Make Breastfeeding Compatible with Family Life

"I don't know how to help my wife
breastfeed our baby."

—DAN

I t is not always a mother who calls my home office requesting breast-feeding help; sometimes the call comes from a new father. I clearly remember a call from Dan, a new father who requested a "personal training" appointment for his wife, Megan. At over six feet tall and three hundred pounds, it was impossible not to notice that Dan was a big man when he opened the door and welcomed me into their home. While I worked with Megan and baby Derik, Dan sat on the edge of the sofa drinking a protein shake and offering encouragement to his wife and son. "You are making great strides, and the two of you are go-ing the distance today." As our visit drew to a close, I learned that Dan was the coach of a winning football team. Megan and Derik continued to breastfeed, and Dan continued to boost the morale of his home team. Without a doubt, Dan, Megan, and Derik are a winning breast-feeding team.

HOW CAN MY PARTNER HELP ME
SUCCESSFULLY BREASTFEED?

Although breastfeeding is women's work, it is a family affair. It is a fact that mothers have a much better chance of breastfeeding success when they have the support of their partner and family.[1] Some new fathers, like Dan, have a knack for providing their wife with the right words of encouragement at the right time. Other dads may feel helpless watching their wife struggle through breastfeeding difficulty. I have witnessed otherwise competent, accomplished men become nearly immobilized by fatherhood because they don't know how to help their wife. Yet, new fathers are in a unique position to make concrete contributions to the breastfeeding process.

For starters, dads can promote togetherness. Keeping a mother and baby in close physical proximity makes breastfeeding possible. Your partner's help is vital if your baby is born by cesarean section, in which case, you will need help caring for your baby and getting physically comfortable enough to breastfeed. In the face of breastfeeding difficulty, a father can further support the breastfeeding process by contacting a lactation consultant or renting a breast pump.

A new baby can never have too much love or attention. A dad can easily comfort his baby between feedings by holding the baby in the skin-to-skin position. I have taught many nervous fathers how to hold and carry their baby in a sling. One dad made a morning ritual of walking in the neighborhood with his son snuggled in a sling. Another new father carried his daughter around the house in a sling. He observed her hunger signals and promptly returned his daughter to his wife to breastfeed whenever she was hungry. Many fathers yearn for the opportunity to forge a close relationship with their new baby but become discouraged because their baby cries whenever they try to hold him or her. If this is your situation, it may be that your baby is hungry and needs to be breastfed. Hold your baby wrapped in a blanket after a feeding. Try walking around with your baby and chances are your baby will instantly settle into your arms.

CAN MY PARTNER FEED OUR BABY?

After spending time in the homes of hundreds of new families, I have come to the conclusion that breastfeeding can't help but flourish in the presence of love and affection. Audra and Pierre stand out in my memory as a couple whose breastfeeding success was a manifestation of their love for each other. I was working with Audra and her daughter Nicola when Pierre returned from the grocery store. After setting the bags down in the kitchen, he came into the living room and balanced himself on the arm of the sofa where Audra was breastfeeding Nicola. Pierre leaned over his wife, kissed her on the lips, and lightly stroked her breast above where Nicola was feeding. Next, he whispered words of encouragement. Nourished by her husband's love, Audra blossomed, and the feeding went very well.

Being with them, I felt drawn in by their love. Looking back, I believe Pierre and Audra's genuine affection for each other carried them through their breastfeeding difficulties. Pierre did not physically feed his daughter that afternoon, but by loving Audra, he made a powerful contribution to her ability to breastfeed. Therefore, his love indirectly fed his daughter.

Pierre did not feel the need to feed Nicola in order to bond with her. He was content to hold Nicola and support Audra's breastfeeding efforts. More often than not, the dads whom I work with are anxious to feed their baby. I have met dads who want so badly to participate in the act of feeding their baby that if biology allowed, I believe they would breastfeed their baby themselves!

Dale, a new father, felt that he wouldn't bond with his son Paul until he fed him. Dale's wife, Alma, was breastfeeding Paul. Dale asked when he could introduce an occasional bottle of Alma's breast milk to Paul. I advised Dale to wait until breastfeeding was well established before giving a bottle to Paul. This may take several weeks or a few months. Of course, when bottle-feeding a breastfed baby, it is always preferable to use breast milk.

During my consultation with Dale and Alma, we devised a plan that would enable Dale to feed his son a bottle of breast milk each evening. Alma was willing to use a breast pump each morning. She then saved the pumped milk for Dale to give Paul later that day. This routine worked well for the family. After work, Dale rushed home so that he could hold and feed his son.

When bottle-feeding a breastfed baby, be aware that bottles have the potential to disrupt your baby's ability to breastfeed. If this occurs, simply stop the bottles for a while. If you want, you can always try to reintroduce a bottle later. Many breastfed babies will drink a bottle very quickly to keep up with the flow from the artificial nipple. You can slow the fast flow by pacing your baby's feeding. To do this, hold the bottle down a bit so that there is a visible air line with your milk in the bottle nipple. Swallowing some air will not harm your baby. You can simply burp your baby after the feeding is finished.

Baby Lillian had two mothers to shower her with love and affection. Rosalyn and Sue had been together since graduate school, and when Rosalyn gave birth to Lillian, their dream of becoming parents became a reality. Rosalyn was exclusively breastfeeding Lillian, and the couple did not want to introduce pacifiers or bottles. I suggested to Sue that if she wanted she could occasionally put Lillian to her breast. Although Sue wasn't making milk, her breast would still calm and comfort her daughter. When I later spoke with the family, Sue shared with me that she nursed Lillian and was able to keep her happy long enough for Rosalyn to take an important phone call.

HOW DO I BREASTFEED MY BABY WHEN I HAVE A TODDLER?

I was happy to hear that my client Gwen had become a mother for the second time. Gwen found that breastfeeding her second baby, Millie, was easier than it had been with her first baby, Michael. Michael was now two years old and had stopped breastfeeding a while before. Gwen was concerned because Michael seemed to have a renewed curiosity about breastfeeding. Gwen wasn't sure how to best handle her son's interest in breastfeeding.

I pointed out to Gwen that it wasn't all that long ago that Michael enjoyed a breastfeeding relationship. Seeing his infant sister breastfeed reminded Michael of the closeness that he once shared with his mother. To satisfy his natural curiosity, I suggested that Gwen provide Michael with some of her expressed breast milk in her son's favorite cup. Michael eagerly accepted the cup, and after walking with the cup clasped between his hands, to Gwen's surprise, Michael returned the cup saying that he no longer wanted "mommy milk." Michael's curiosity about breastfeeding and breast milk had been satisfied.

Sometimes breastfeeding a second baby provides a mother with a unique opportunity to heal from past breastfeeding difficulty. I met Alex shortly after her second son, Ryan, was born. Alex regretted that she had given up breastfeeding her first son, Johnny, when he was just days old. During our consultation, I could tell by her tears that Alex was still grieving over her inability to provide Johnny, now eighteen months old, with the benefits of breastfeeding. There was an obvious solution to the sadness that Alex was experiencing.

I suggested to Alex that she had more than enough breast milk to fully breastfeed Ryan and if she wished she could regularly provide Johnny with her milk in his "sippy" cup. Of course, Alex could not go back in time, but she could look forward to providing Johnny with the gifts of her milk now. Alex embraced this idea. At no time did pumping fresh milk for Johnny impede Alex's ability to exclusively breastfeed Ryan. Both children were thriving, and instead of looking back with regret, Alex looked forward to her future as a breastfeeding mother.

Providing your toddler or older child with fresh or refrigerated breast milk is especially beneficial during illness. The antibodies in your breast milk can aid your child's recovery. Some mothers breastfeed an older child and a baby together. This practice is called *tandem nursing*. By continuing to breastfeed, an older child is not displaced from the breast by a new brother or sister. This can ease sibling rivalry as an older child becomes accustomed to the unfamiliar role of big sister or big brother.

IS BREASTFEEDING COMPATIBLE WITH ROMANCE?

Jill confided that sex with her husband was different since having a baby, "We had great sex, but now instead of pleasurable, sex is uncomfortable." Due to medical complications, Jill spent most of her pregnancy on bed rest, during which time the doctor advised her to abstain from sexual activity. Jill and her husband were relieved when their son Jared was born healthy and near his due date. Jill had been exclusively breastfeeding Jared who was now two months old. After Jill's six-week postpartum check-up, the doctor cleared her for sex. Unfortunately, the romantic encounter that Jill and her husband had been waiting for turned out to be somewhat disappointing. Jill was relieved to hear that many of my clients describe similar experiences when resuming a sexual relationship with their partner.

Breastfeeding and mothering hormones can inhibit a new mother's enjoyment of sexual intercourse. After having a baby, breastfeeding hormones as well as the lack of the hormone estrogen cause a mother's vagina to remain dry during sexual stimulation.[2] This can make intercourse uncomfortable, even painful. Traditionally, new mothers are told to abstain from sexual intercourse until given the green light from their obstetrician at their six-week postpartum check-up. Each mother recovers from childbirth at her own pace. For a mother recovering from an episiotomy, tearing, or cesarean section, six weeks may be too early to resume sexual relations. On a hormonal level, your sexuality will eventually be restored, and your body will once again welcome and respond to lovemaking. In the meantime, I recommend that new mothers use an over-the-counter personal lubricant to make intercourse more comfortable.

In practical terms, caring for a new baby may leave both parents too physically exhausted to do anything but sleep in bed. Adjusting to having a baby in the house can strain even the happiest of relationships and cause marital resentments to pile up faster than dirty laundry. As a new mother, you may not feel particularly sexy wearing a nursing bra all day, and you may not fit into your favorite clothes that once made you feel good about your body. All these reasons make it difficult for couples to shift gears from parents to romantic partners. During this transition time, find out what your partner needs to feel loved and appreciated and, in return, communicate what it is that you need to feel nurtured.

CAN I BECOME PREGNANT WHILE BREASTFEEDING?

Hillary had a postpartum check-up at her obstetrician's office. After a pelvic exam, the doctor declared that she had healed from childbirth and gave Hillary the go-ahead to resume a sexual relationship with her husband. Because Hillary was breastfeeding her six-week-old baby, Josh, she was not sure what birth control method to use. Hillary did not want to become pregnant right away, and her husband did not want to wear a condom. For these reasons, the obstetrician gave Hillary a prescription for the mini-pill.

Before filling the prescription, Hillary called to ask me if it was possible to become pregnant while breastfeeding Josh. Under certain conditions breastfeeding can act as very effective birth control. To determine if breastfeeding would protect Hillary from becoming pregnant, I needed to ask about the nature of her breastfeeding relationship with Josh. Hillary stated that she exclusively breastfed Josh both during the day and at night. Josh did not receive any formula or other supplements, and Hillary had not yet gotten a menstrual period. Hillary met all three criteria for the lactational amenorrhea form of birth control; she was exclusively breastfeeding a baby under the age of six months, and she had not gotten her period. Hillary had only a 1 to 2 percent chance of becoming pregnant at this time.

Hillary was surprised to learn that she could lessen her chances of becoming pregnant simply by breastfeeding Josh. The lactational amenorrhea method (LAM) is based on the simple fact that the hormones that regulate breastfeeding inhibit a woman's fertility. It's as if a mother's body becomes too preoccupied with breastfeeding her baby to become pregnant again. LAM is a reliable method of natural family planning for mothers who have not gotten a menstrual period and who are exclusively breastfeeding a baby younger than six months old.[3]

If, for any reason, one of the three criteria for LAM is no longer being met, it can no longer be relied on to prevent pregnancy. For example, if a sexually active mother begins to regularly supplement her two-month-old breastfed baby with bottles of formula or pumped breast milk, then it is necessary for her to use another method of birth control if she does not wish to become pregnant. When choosing a method of birth control, it is important to recognize that some methods of birth control support the continuation of breastfeeding more than others.

A woman's partner can support breastfeeding by wearing a condom or having a vasectomy if no further pregnancies are planned. A breastfeeding mother can be fitted for a diaphragm or intrauterine device, use spermicide, or have a tubal ligation for permanent pregnancy prevention. These methods do not contain hormones, and, therefore, do not interfere with breastfeeding. If nonhormonal contraceptive methods are not workable for you and your partner, then birth control that contains hormones is the next option.

The problem with commonly prescribed hormonal birth control methods like mini-pills and injectables is that it is unclear whether these methods disrupt breastfeeding by suppressing a mother's milk supply.[4] The greatest concern is when these methods are given in the first days after childbirth before breastfeeding is fully established. In my professional experience, injectable birth control and the mini-pill both lower a mother's milk supply. Mini-pills, injectables, and birth control implants contain progestin, and to avoid potential milk supply problems, it is recommended that new mothers wait until breastfeeding is well established before starting these birth control methods.[5] Even so, I have had clients experience the side effect of low milk supply after receiving injectable birth control at their six-week postpartum appointment. Traditional birth control pills that contain the hormone estrogen are not recommended until after six months postpartum.

DO I HAVE TO STOP BREASTFEEDING IF I WANT TO BECOME PREGNANT?

Theo had just celebrated her daughter Ellie's first birthday. No longer a baby, Ellie had grown into a happy easygoing little girl. Although Ellie was busy exploring the world and learning to walk, she still enjoyed breastfeeding, especially before going to bed at night. Theo and her husband wanted to provide Ellie with a brother or sister. Theo wondered if she needed to completely stop breastfeeding before she could conceive another baby.

Because Theo breastfed Ellie sporadically during the day and once at bedtime, it is unlikely that her breastfeeding relationship would interfere with her ability to become pregnant. Theo had recently resumed a regular menstrual cycle, a sure signal that her fertility was returning. Breastfeeding is not contraindicated during normal pregnancy. However, ovulation and subsequent pregnancy may cause nipple sensitivity that can make breastfeeding unbearably painful. Additionally, breastfeeding naturally causes uterine contractions that can be alarming to a pregnant mother. Finally, pregnancy will alter the taste and lower the volume of your breast milk. These changes can cause an older child to stop breastfeeding all on his or her own.

HOW CAN I FIT ROMANCE INTO MY LIFE?

Sexual feelings exist on a continuum. Courtships and honeymoons are traditionally a time when lovers shower each other with physical affection. Although you still need affection after having a baby, it is natural and normal for you to experience a decrease in your need for sex. Recognize this as being a temporary situation. Although caring for your new baby is your first priority, it is also important to tend to your partner's need for physical and emotional love. Breastfeeding is compatible with family life and a romantic relationship.

Recognize that your body needs time to recover

You may not feel ready to resume a sexual relationship for quite some time after childbirth. The traditional six-week waiting period may not be enough time to heal from a difficult birth, episiotomy, or a cesarean section. Be patient. Each woman recovers at her own pace. Recognize that the hormones that enable you to breastfeed and care for your new baby may dampen your sex drive. For the time being, you may not feel the need to have sex. The love you feel for your partner may be as strong as ever, but your motivation to express your love in a physical way may be decreased. If you hesitate to resume intercourse for fear that it will be uncomfortable, plan to use a store-bought lubricant designed for that purpose. You may be surprised to hear that some of my clients have told me that after a few months, breastfeeding actually increased rather than decreased their sex drive.

Shift your role to make romance

You may not find your new role as a mother particularly sexy, but I'll bet your partner finds you as desirable as ever. Caring for a baby is an all-consuming endeavor. In order to feel romantic, it may help you to take intentional steps that lead you toward an amorous encounter with your partner. To feel sexy, change your clothes, take off your nursing bra, and put on your favorite perfume. Clear away the diapers (especially dirty ones) and baby clothes from your bed. Have dinner and dessert delivered from your favorite restaurant and enjoy a meal with your partner. Spend a few minutes talking and listening to each other. Enjoy being together both emotionally and physically.

Review your options for birth control

One of the benefits of breastfeeding is that you may be able to enjoy natural family planning. LAM is based on the fact that frequent breastfeeding both during the day and at night suppresses a mother's fertility. It is unlikely that a breastfeeding mother will become pregnant if she has not gotten a menstrual period, is exclusively breastfeeding, and her baby is under six months of age. If one of these criteria is not met, then another birth control method is needed to prevent pregnancy. Birth control methods that do not contain hormones are the most compatible with breastfeeding. The mini-pill and injectable birth control contain progestin and are anecdotally known to lower milk supply in some mothers. Birth control pills that contain estrogen will suppress milk supply and should not be used until at least six months after childbirth.

SUMMARY OF BREASTFEEDING ABCs

Breastfeeding is compatible with modern family life. New fathers play an important role in making breastfeeding work by supporting their wife's breastfeeding efforts. Some dads feel a strong desire to feed their baby as a means of bonding with their new son or daughter. It is preferable to wait until breastfeeding is firmly established and to use only pumped breast milk when giving your baby a bottle. Older siblings may become curious about breastfeeding and want to try some of your breast milk. Feel free to offer your expressed milk in a cup to your toddler or child. Take your time when it comes to romance. If you had a passionate love life before your baby was born, chances are good that you and your partner will have a passionate relationship in the future.

A. AFFECTION

Breastfeeding flourishes in an environment filled with love and affection. New dads can support their partner's breastfeeding efforts simply by offering an encouraging word, a hug, or a kiss at just the right time. Your new baby can never have too much love and physical affection. Have your partner hold your baby after a feeding. Many new fathers feel frustrated and helpless when holding their crying baby. It is likely that the baby is crying out of hunger. This can be avoided by holding your baby after instead of before a feeding.

B. BIRTH CONTROL

Explore all of your options when considering birth control. LAM is a reliable form of natural family planning. A mother can utilize LAM if she has not gotten her menstrual period and is exclusively breastfeeding a baby younger than six months of age. If these conditions are not met, then an additional birth control method is needed to prevent pregnancy. Nonhormonal methods of birth control are considered the most compatible with breastfeeding. Examples of such methods include condoms, diaphragms, and spermicides. The mini-pill and injectable birth control are hormonal forms of birth control. Currently, it is unclear whether these methods lower a mother's milk supply. There is plenty of anecdotal evidence that mini-pills and injectable birth control suppress milk supply especially when given in the early postpartum period.

C. CONCEIVE

It is possible to become pregnant while breastfeeding. The resumption of a regular menstrual period signals that your fertility is returning. If you want to conceive another baby and are still breastfeeding, it may not be necessary for you to completely end your current breastfeeding relationship. Breastfeeding before naps or before bedtime probably won't interfere with your ability to become pregnant. Nipple soreness is common during ovulation and pregnancy. If you continue breastfeeding after conceiving another baby, the taste of your breast milk will change, and your milk supply will naturally decrease. These changes may prompt some nursing toddlers to stop breastfeeding all together. However, it is completely safe to continue breastfeeding during a normal pregnancy.

CHAPTER SEVENTEEN

Combining Breastfeeding with Your Career

> "I love the fact that he gets my
> milk while I am working."
> —MELANIE

Melanie worked for several years as a graphic artist for a small advertising company. After her son Sean was born, Melanie called me for advice on combining motherhood and breast-feeding with her career. Melanie was the first employee to return from maternity leave and request time and privacy during the day to pump breast milk. The problem was that Melanie's boss balked at the notion of one of his employees expressing breast milk during the work-day. He and his wife had formula fed their two children. Melanie did not want to formula feed Sean when she went back to work. Breastfeeding Sean had always been a pleasure, and the pediatrician said that Sean was growing perfectly.

During our consultation, I explained that to maintain a full milk sup-ply and provide fresh milk for Sean at day care, Melanie would need to express her milk with an electric pump two or three times during the workday. Since a private office was not available, Melanie purchased a portable screen to use around her desk and planned to pump during cof-fee and lunch breaks so that the flow of office work was not disrupted.

Over the course of several discussions with her boss, Melanie patiently explained that her milk would protect her son from common illness while he was in day care, therefore lessening the likelihood that she would miss work caring for a sick child. Melanie's boss became more supportive, and, thanks to her persistence, Melanie paved the way for one of her coworkers to continue breastfeeding after she returned from maternity leave.

IS BREASTFEEDING COMPATIBLE WITH MY CAREER?

I remember visiting Lynn when her daughter was barely five days old. Lynn ran a very successful business that employed more than one hundred people. Over the course of our consultation, Lynn described how productive her workday was, who was running the office in her absence, and what needed to be accomplished when she returned to work. When I attempted to shift the tide of Lynn's attention toward holding and breastfeeding her infant daughter, she once again became swept up in the drama of her career. Six weeks later, Lynn was back working full-time, and her baby was placed in full-time day care. Breastfeeding fell by the wayside.

I am saddened whenever I come across a new mother like Lynn who is unable to grasp the significance of her mothering role. Motherhood transforms every woman's usual workday into a lifetime commitment of caring for her child. Value the investment of time that you spend mothering your baby. If your future includes employment, focus your present energy on establishing a fulfilling breastfeeding relationship with your baby.

Breastfeeding is compatible with working outside the home. The key to combining breastfeeding with your career is to build a firm breastfeeding foundation with your baby. To do this, spend as much time as possible holding and breastfeeding your baby while you are home on maternity leave. For the time being, forget about the office and focus on fostering a strong successful breastfeeding relationship. You and your baby will be able to restructure breastfeeding when you are ready to relaunch your career.

IS IT IMPORTANT TO CONTINUE BREASTFEEDING?

Many new mothers feel they must end their breastfeeding relationship because they are returning to work.[1] When I met Eliza, she made it clear that she wasn't going to continue breastfeeding after her maternity leave was over. She found the idea of pumping at work unappealing and too time consuming. As her maternity leave drew to a close, Eliza quickly switched Dominic to formula and bottles.

By the time Dominic was four months old, Eliza was working full-time, and Dominic had transitioned to full-time day care. Initially, the arrangement seemed to work, but within three weeks, Dominic began to run high fevers and developed infections in both ears. Dominic was unable to fully recover from one bout of illness before contracting another infection. In addition to the pediatrician, Dominic needed to see a specialist for his ear problems. Because of Dominic's medical condition, Eliza missed many days of work, and several important meetings went on without her. Eliza wondered if Dominic would be happier and in better health if she had continued breastfeeding instead of formula feeding when she returned to work.

As you contemplate returning to work, consider how important your breast milk is to your baby's well-being. While you work, your milk will be there to nourish and protect your baby from common illnesses. If your baby does become ill while in a daycare setting, the antibodies your baby receives while breastfeeding will aid your baby's recovery. Best of all, breastfeeding your baby after work enables the two of you to quickly and effortlessly reconnect after being apart.

SHOULD I STOP BREASTFEEDING TO MAKE DAY CARE EASIER?

Addie, a working mother, wasn't sure whether to continue breastfeeding her six-month-old son, Tommy, or to stop breastfeeding altogether. Tommy cried every morning when Addie dropped him off at day care on the way to work. When she returned at the end of the day, Tommy was hungry and would breastfeed voraciously. The daycare provider consistently reported that Tommy wouldn't take much from the bottles of pumped breast milk Addie packed for him each day.

Back at home, nighttime with Tommy wasn't easy either. When Addie tried to put Tommy in his crib at night, he would thrash about and cry frantically. He seldom slept for more than two consecutive hours before waking up to breastfeed. The pediatrician attributed Tommy's behavior to breastfeeding. The doctor told Addie that once she stopped breastfeeding, Tommy would stop crying at day care and begin sleeping all night. Addie wasn't sure what she should do. Both Tommy's daycare provider and his doctor wanted Tommy to be formula fed, yet breastfeeding made Tommy happy, and Addie didn't want to stop when the rest of life was so stressful.

Addie's mothering instinct was right. Tommy needed breastfeeding more than ever. The benefits to his physical and emotional well-being are irreplaceable. To cope with separation during the day and crying at night, I recommended that Addie take a more compassionate approach than what her babysitter and pediatrician recommended. I explained to Addie that it is not unusual or abnormal for Tommy to cry after being dropped off in the morning. Breastfeeding Tommy at this time could help to lessen his separation anxiety. As Tommy grows and develops, this natural anxiety should lessen.

The fact that Tommy consumed very little of his bottles during the day worried his daycare provider. I explained to Addie that Tommy made up for his low intake at day care by breastfeeding frequently when he was reunited with her. Some breastfed babies like Tommy naturally regulate themselves so that they take very little during daycare hours and consume the bulk of their feeding when with their mother. To work with Tommy's feeding pattern, I suggested that Addie request the daycare provider offer Tommy smaller snacks of pumped breast milk or his favorite solid foods at frequent intervals throughout the day.

Finally, I advised Addie to utilize her breastfeeding relationship with Tommy to make nighttime a bonding experience instead of an unpleasant struggle. The message behind Tommy's relentless crying was crystal clear. He needed the reassurance of being close to Addie at night. Addie could foster this closeness by keeping Tommy near her at night and breastfeeding from the side-lying position so they could rest together. Contrary to what the daycare provider and doctor thought, I believe breastfeeding was what Tommy needed most. Putting an end to breastfeeding would increase rather than decrease Tommy's separation anxiety and lead to more crying.

HOW DO I PREPARE TO REENTER THE WORKPLACE?

The first step to preparing to reenter the workplace as a breastfeeding mother is to build a strong breastfeeding relationship with your baby. My clients who plan to work outside the home often ask me what they can do to get ready for work when their baby is just a few days old. My answer is always the same: continue to hold and breastfeed your baby. Take as much maternity leave as your career and personal finances allow. Use this time to recover from childbirth and establish a breastfeeding relationship with your new baby. After you have developed a full milk supply and your baby is at least one month old, you will be ready to explore the question of how to comfortably return to the workforce while breastfeeding. Consider the following four points as you begin to plan your strategy for returning to work.

Your work hours

The particular details of your plan will depend in large part on whether you are working full-time or part-time hours. Without a doubt, it is easier to combine mothering, work, and breastfeeding on a part-time work schedule; however, it is possible to continue breastfeeding while working full-time. Take into consideration how long it will take you to commute back and forth to work. One of my clients changed jobs to work closer to home. Her new job saved her a full hour of travel time each day. Another of my clients chose to work longer hours, but all of her work hours were spent in her home office. This arrangement allowed her the opportunity to breastfeed her son for most of his feedings. Consider all of your career options. A simple change in your work schedule may provide you the time and flexibility you need to continue breastfeeding.

Your work space

Visit your work space and touch base with your coworkers during your maternity leave. Use this opportunity to scout out a suitable place to pump your milk when you return to work. Ideally, this space should be private, have a door that you can close, and have an electrical outlet for your pump. It is also helpful to have access to a sink where you can wash your hands and rinse out your collection kit. The space should be available for at least two fifteen- to twenty-minute intervals during your workday. Keep in mind that a bathroom does not qualify as a suitable place to express milk for your baby. Some states, such as Connecticut, have passed legislation protecting a mother's right to pump her breast milk while working. The legislation calls on larger businesses to provide space and opportunity for breastfeeding mothers to pump and store milk for their babies.[2]

Your baby and bottles

Jodie was nearing the end of her sixteen-week maternity leave, and her daughter Liz wouldn't take a bottle. Jodie tried putting her pumped breast milk into four different types of bottles, but Liz wouldn't accept any of them. It seemed that the more Jodie and her husband tried the bottle, the more Liz would turn away and cry. Adding to the sense of urgency was Jodie's daycare provider, who told her that Liz would have to be able to bottle-feed to stay at the daycare center.

Don't panic if your baby has difficulty drinking from a bottle. Choose a bottle with a broad base around the nipple such as the Avent bottle with a newborn-size nipple. Gently encourage your baby to take hold of the bottle nipple and offer your baby a small amount of your pumped breast milk from the bottle. Try offering the bottle while walking around with your baby in a sling or infant front pack. Never force or push a bottle nipple into your baby's mouth; this will frighten your baby. Practice bottle-feeding when your baby is not overly hungry.

I have known a few babies who would not easily accept a bottle. Luckily, most babies who have difficulty bottle-feeding can easily finger feed from the tubing of an SNS attached to a caregiver's index finger. Another option is to have your daycare provider feed your baby breast milk with a cup or a spoon. It's helpful if your daycare provider is open to trying these methods.

Your daycare provider

Find a daycare provider who will be a breastfeeding ally. Whether you plan to use a large daycare center, try a home-based day care, or hire a nanny, be sure that they are willing to support your breastfeeding relationship. Your babysitter should be comfortable warming bottles of breast milk and be willing to offer your baby a smaller feeding near pick-up time so that your baby will be ready to breastfeed when reunited with you. The daycare provider should not overfeed your baby from a bottle. A babysitter caring for one of my client's babies switched the baby to a larger bottle nipple and proceeded to feed the baby twelve ounces in twenty minutes, which is more than twice a normal feeding.

As you investigate child-care options, consider the location of the daycare center. Having your baby in a daycare center close to your office or, better yet, on your work site gives you the opportunity to breastfeed your baby at lunchtime. This is a huge advantage to you, your baby, and your breastfeeding relationship. If you can't leave the work site to breastfeed, consider asking a family member to bring your baby to work for a feeding during the day.

HOW DO I STORE MY MILK BEFORE
GOING BACK TO WORK?

Josephina was so determined to provide her son Gabby with a full supply of breast milk when she returned to work that she decided to get a head start. In addition to breastfeeding Gabby, Josephina began to pump and store her milk soon after Gabby was born. All of this extra pumping resulted in a tremendous breast milk imbalance. After a while, Josephina regularly produced enough milk to feed twins. Her breasts were overfull and she found herself in a perpetual state of discomfort. Gabby was equally unhappy because he was unable to manage his mother's overflow of breast milk during feeding.

Josephina's mistake was that she started pumping and storing her milk before her body had the opportunity to learn how much milk Gabby needed. Before regularly storing your milk, it is important to allow your body to naturally adjust to your baby's needs. Take time to enter into a state of harmony and balance before you begin the process of preparing for work.

Start regularly pumping and storing your milk a few weeks before you plan to return to work. The best time to pump is after breastfeeding your baby in the morning. Pump both breasts for a few minutes and store the milk in specially made breast milk storage bags. Write the date on the bag before you pour your milk into the bag. You can combine milk from the left and right breasts before storing it in two- or four-ounce portions in the freezer. Your milk can be stored in the freezer for six months. Fresh refrigerated breast milk is good for a week. Thaw bags of frozen breast milk in a bowl of hot water or under running water. Do not microwave breast milk and do not refreeze thawed milk. Use any thawed milk within twenty-four hours. Finally, do not add fresh pumped milk to frozen breast milk and attempt to refreeze it.

Besides building a stored supply of breast milk, another advantage of regularly pumping before returning to work is that you will become acclimated to the feeling of your breast pump. In order to successfully use your breast pump at work, it is important to first become comfortable pumping at home. To keep your supply strong while you are at work, it is necessary to pump with a hospital-grade double electric breast pump such as the Pump in Style by Medela or Purely Yours by Ameda. Using a hospital-grade pump will stimulate your breastfeeding hormones more effectively than a manual or non–hospital-grade pump.[3]

Believe it or not, there is more to using a breast pump than meets the eye. To get your milk flowing, your body must believe that you are breast-feeding your baby. Think about your baby and imagine breastfeeding while pumping. Some moms find it helpful to smell a shirt recently worn by their baby or to look at their baby's picture while pumping. Cover the collection bottles with a baby blanket to avoid becoming preoccupied or worried about how much milk you are able to pump. Pumping for ten minutes should be sufficient for most mothers to collect their breast milk. Be careful to keep the suction on a low or medium setting and don't press the cones of the collection kit too hard against your breasts.

HOW DO I MAINTAIN MY MILK SUPPLY WHILE WORKING?

Whether you plan to work part-time or full-time, the principles of com-bining breastfeeding and employment are the same. The idea is to breast-feed as often as possible when you and your baby are together and to pump at select intervals when you are apart. Individualize the steps that follow to fit your unique work situation. Being a breastfeeding mom in the workforce takes effort, but at the end of each day, you can be proud knowing that you are providing your baby with the gift of your milk while you are apart.

Balancing breastfeeding and pumping

Plan to breastfeed your baby before leaving for work. If possible, pump both breasts immediately afterward. Your baby can be fed the fresh milk from the pumping session later in the morning. During a traditional eight-hour workday, plan to pump two or three times or about every three hours. To maintain a full milk supply, it is necessary to pump both breasts at the same time for about ten minutes. Store your pumped breast milk in a cooler with blue ice or in the refrigerator. The milk that you pump at work can be fed to your baby the following day. If possible, pump once more after breastfeeding your baby in the evening before going to bed. Breastfeeding your baby whenever the two of you are together will invigorate your milk supply.

After using your breast pump, simply rinse the collection kit with hot soapy water (not the tubing) or clean it with wipes designed for that purpose. For the sake of convenience, consider investing in two collection kits that you can wash at the end of the day. It is not necessary to boil or sterilize your collection kit to the point of disintegration.

Feeding your baby at day care

The amount of breast milk that you leave for your baby in your absence depends on how long you will be apart and your baby's feeding pattern. I recommend preparing a combination of larger amounts and a few smaller snack-size servings of breast milk. Packing a variety of amounts lessens the likelihood that your breast milk will be wasted. While you are working, your baby may consume less than usual and wait to be with you to breastfeed. Conversely, your baby may consume artificially high volumes of breast milk from the bottle. To keep this from happening, provide your babysitter with appropriate amounts of your milk in each bottle and use a newborn-size nipple. Ask whoever is feeding your baby to pace the feeding so that the flow is not too fast.

If you have cultivated a full supply of breast milk before going back to work, then chances are good that you will be able to maintain your supply. If breastfeeding is going well, it is not necessary to formula feed your baby prior to beginning work. There is no benefit to unnecessarily exposing your breastfed baby to formula. If in the future the situation arises that requires you to augment your breast milk with formula, you can introduce formula at that time. In the meantime, have faith in your ability to combine motherhood and breastfeeding with your career.

SUMMARY OF BREASTFEEDING ABCs

It is possible to continue breastfeeding your baby after going back to work. To do this, you must first build a strong breastfeeding relationship with your baby. After giving birth, concentrate on becoming comfortable caring for and breastfeeding your baby. Don't make the mistake of intentionally pumping and storing your milk too early. Allow your body the opportunity to naturally adjust to how much milk your baby needs. This takes at least a month. Once you and your baby have achieved a state of harmony, you can begin pumping and storing milk once a day in preparation for returning to work. Pumping once in the morning will give you plenty of milk without disturbing the balance of your supply. While at work, it is important to regularly pump with a hospital-grade double electric breast pump to preserve your milk supply.

A. ADJUST

Going back to work is an adjustment for you and your baby. Continuing to breastfeed can ease this adjustment. Breastfeeding your baby enables you to maintain your special bond and allows you to effortlessly reconnect after being apart. Some babies automatically adjust their feeding pattern to match their mother's work schedule so that they take very little from their caregiver and breastfeed often when with their mother. Another advantage of continuing to breastfeed is that the consistency of breastfeeding will ease your baby's adjustment to day care.

B. BOTTLE FEEDING

If you plan to go back to work, gently introduce your baby to bottle-feeding after breastfeeding is well established. Choose a bottle with a broad base around the nipple. Offer your baby the bottle containing some of your breast milk when your baby is not overly hungry. Don't panic if your baby has difficulty bottle-feeding. Try offering the bottle while walking around with your baby in a sling or infant front pack. Never force the bottle into your baby's mouth and pace the feeding so your baby is not overwhelmed by the fast flow of the bottle. If your baby has difficulty bottle-feeding, try cup feeding, spoon feeding, or finger feeding.

C. CAREER

Breastfeeding is compatible with your career. To combine working with breastfeeding, you will need to first establish a strong breastfeeding relationship with your baby. To maintain your milk supply and provide your baby with breast milk, you will need to regularly use a breast pump during your workday. Plan to breastfeed your baby whenever you are together. This will preserve your breastfeeding relationship and invigorate your milk supply. While working, you will need to pump both breasts together for ten minutes with an electric breast pump. Ideally, this should be done every three hours. Use that milk to feed your baby at day care the following day or freeze it for future use.

CHAPTER EIGHTEEN

When Is the Right Time to Wean?

"I want to know how to stop
breastfeeding when I am ready."

—RILEY

had been working with Riley and Nikko in their home for about an hour when Riley told me that her plan was to breastfeed her son for six months and then wean him. With that goal in mind, she asked me how to plan for weaning. Under the circumstances, it seemed an odd question for a new mother to ask. Riley was just becoming accustomed to breastfeeding and Nikko was barely one week old. Yet Riley's question did not surprise me. Nearly every mother who requests my help beginning a breastfeeding relationship wants to know how and when it will end.

From the perspective of having worked with hundreds of new mothers and their babies, I view breastfeeding as a transformative journey rather than a series of random feedings. Although it is not a bad idea to look forward in anticipation of arriving at your destination of weaning, I recommend my clients keep an open-ended ticket instead of booking a nonrefundable round trip. Along the way, you may find sight-seeing irresistible. You may be unexpectedly drawn down a cobblestone walkway or into an aromatic garden of yellow roses. One misty morning you may be awakened by the call of seagulls circling above a distant beach beckoning you to sit on the sand and observe the shifting tides.

Sure, your travel agent booked you for a three-month stay, but with all of these scenic diversions, you may need another three months to reach your chosen destination. Unlike the gasoline in your car or seats on a crowded airplane, breast milk never runs dry, and there are no restrictions to breast-feeding. You and your baby are allowed to continue traveling together for as long as you want.

HOW DOES WEANING BEGIN?

Weaning begins when your baby is regularly consuming foods or liquids in place of breast milk. Because your breast milk provides complete nutrition for the first six months of your baby's life, other foods and drinks are not necessary before this time.[1] Ideally, weaning occurs gradually when your baby is developmentally ready to eat solid foods and drink from a cup. Over time, your milk production will adjust as your baby eats more food and breastfeeds less often. When both of you are ready to move on to another phase of your relationship, breastfeeding will fade into the background and will no longer be the focus of your relationship.

WILL QUICKLY WEANING ENCOURAGE
MY BABY TO EAT MORE FOOD?

Tina took her daughter Morgan to the pediatrician for a routine visit. Morgan was just over six months old and had started eating solid foods. In conjunction with regular meals, Morgan breastfed throughout the day and several times during the night. The pediatrician told Tina that Morgan was healthy and growing well. However, she recommended that Tina cut back on breastfeeding so that Morgan would eat larger amounts of food. The pediatrician went on to say that by now, Morgan had gotten all the benefits of breastfeeding and that there was very little to be gained from continuing. Tina wasn't sure what she should do. Morgan clearly enjoyed breastfeeding, and because she was under one year of age, Morgan was too young to drink cow's milk. Tina did not want to feed Morgan formula in place of breast milk.

There is plenty to be gained from continuing to breastfeed after your baby regularly eats meals. Breast milk still provides your baby with essential proteins and nutrients and boosts your baby's immune system. Both the AAP and the World Health Organization (WHO) recognize the value that breastfeeding provides to older babies, and both authorities recommend that mothers continue to breastfeed after introducing their babies to solid foods.[2] The reassurance that breastfeeding provides to your baby may be more important than ever as your baby begins to explore the world and tackle new developmental milestones. Each baby adapts to the experience of eating solid foods at his or her own pace. Abruptly ending a breastfeeding relationship will not necessarily cause a baby to consume more solid food. Additionally, there is no reason for a mother like Tina to begin formula feeding her daughter when she has a plentiful supply of breast milk.

IS THERE A WRONG TIME TO WEAN?

When considering whether to stop breastfeeding, take your own feelings into account. The worst time to wean is when you don't want to but feel pressured to stop breastfeeding from outside influences. Remember that you know your baby best. If your instincts tell you to continue breastfeeding, then breastfeeding is what is right every time.

Marcie wished she had listened to her inner voice when it came to weaning her son Ryan. Initially, breastfeeding seemed to be going well. But by the time Ryan was three months old, he had developed an allergic skin condition and reflux that caused him to vomit large portions of his feedings several times a day. Marcie took Ryan to see a specialist. The doctor prescribed medication to help control Ryan's reflux and recommended that Ryan be fed a special formula. Marcie did not want to stop breastfeeding, but the doctor insisted that the hypoallergenic formula would control Ryan's symptoms.

Against her better judgment, Marcie stopped breastfeeding. A month later, Ryan's reflux was no better on the new formula than it had been when he was breastfed. Marcie missed breastfeeding Ryan and wished she hadn't agreed to give it up so easily. I have personal experience in this area and empathize with Marcie's dilemma. Like Marcie, I was advised by a doctor to stop breastfeeding.

My daughter Miriam was born weighing five pounds, six ounces. She was a small but perfectly healthy baby, and as she grew older she remained small. Despite being breastfed, Miriam weighed only fourteen pounds by her first birthday, far below what was considered normal. Miriam was evaluated by a cadre of specialists at the medical center where I worked. The stern-faced specialists either failed to notice or were unmoved by Miriam's cheerful nature and big smile. A battery of blood tests confirmed that despite her diminutive size, she was healthy. Nonetheless, Miriam was labeled "failure-to-thrive." The diagnosis left me feeling like a failure of a mother. I loved every ounce of my little girl and didn't much care that she was too small to fit onto a standard growth chart. The prescribed treatment plan was painfully simple. I was to stop breastfeeding, and in place of breast milk, Miriam was to consume a high-calorie concoction.

I knew with all my heart that breastfeeding was what Miriam needed most. Although I disagreed with Miriam's medical doctors, I did not dismiss all of their advice. We began a developmental therapy program to help Miriam comfortably adjust to solid food, and, to my surprise, she willingly drank the high-calorie supplement from a cup. Miriam and I went on to breastfeed for another full year, during which time she outgrew that awful failure-to-thrive diagnosis. Today, Miriam is a tall, athletic third grader, and her smile is brighter than ever. Looking back, I am proud that I listened to the voice of my mothering instinct and continued to breastfeed.

WILL MY BABY SELF-WEAN?

Vicki told me that her daughter Tegan had stopped breastfeeding all on her own. When she was eight months old, Tegan seemed to lose interest in breastfeeding, and Vicki began to offer more bottles and cups. Finally, Tegan refused to breastfeed. Now that Vicki was pregnant again, she was hoping that her new baby would breastfeed for a full year. Vicki's experience with Tegan is not uncommon. Many older babies become distracted while breastfeeding and quickly wean when offered an increasing number of feedings from bottles and cups. Habitually sucking on a pacifier can also replace breastfeeding time. If you and your baby are comfortable gradually ending your breastfeeding relationship this way, then you are stopping at the right time. If, on the other hand, your baby is frequently upset and is unable to accept a cup in place of breastfeeding, then your baby may not be ready to wean. Although your baby may readily eat solids and drink from a cup, it is normal for your baby to need the reassurance of breastfeeding before bedtime. Ideally, weaning should happen gradually at a pace that is comfortable for both of you. Complete weaning does not occur overnight.

If your baby suddenly refuses to breastfeed, then your baby could be having a nursing strike. A nursing strike is your baby's way of telling you that something has upset his or her usual routine. For example, your baby may be teething, have an earache, or feel rushed at feeding time. Investigate the events that preceded your baby's refusal to nurse. If nothing is causing your baby physical distress, then it may be that your baby has been given bottles or a pacifier more than usual. Luckily, most nursing strikes are self-limiting and are over within a day or two. In the meantime, it may help to carry your baby close to your body in a sling or front pack. The rhythm of your moving body may comfort and relax your baby enough to begin breastfeeding again. If feeding time has been hectic, your baby may respond to an unhurried feeding in the early morning before the day is fully under way.

CAN I BREASTFEED WHEN MY BABY GETS TEETH?

I have heard many new mothers say they can't imagine breastfeeding when their baby has teeth. Yet, when that first white tooth pokes through your baby's pink gum, you may find that neither one of you is ready to stop breastfeeding. It is understandable to fear being bitten. Knowing what to do if this occurs should calm your anxiety. If your baby accidentally bites your nipple while breastfeeding, quickly pull your baby into your chest. Tell your baby, "No," and end the feeding. Resist the urge to push your baby away from you. This can injure your nipple if your baby hasn't let go. Biting is more likely to occur toward the end of a feeding. If your baby has bitten you in the past, pay attention as the feeding winds down and remove your baby before the biting occurs.

HOW OLD IS TOO OLD TO BREASTFEED?

While driving through Hartford on my way to a consultation, I was listening to a popular radio station. Between songs the disc jockey told a story about a mother who breastfeeds her three-year-old child. The way he criticized the mother's breastfeeding relationship upset me so much that I exited the highway and drove to the radio station. Once at the radio station, I waited in the lobby to meet the disc jockey. After some time, I was able to give him my business card and politely explain that in many cultures breastfeeding an older child is not considered unusual or aberrant behavior. The disc jockey agreed to call me if he had any questions about breastfeeding in the future.

As my experience at the radio station illustrates, extended breastfeeding is a misunderstood and emotionally charged issue. The notion of breastfeeding a baby over a certain age is downright bizarre to some mothers. The exact age at which a baby becomes a child who is too old to breastfeed varies from one mother to the next. I found this out while teaching a hospital-based class for expectant parents. I nearly lost control of the group when I began discussing the benefits breastfeeding provides to older children. A mother in the back of the room didn't believe that anyone would breastfeed a three- or four-year-old. Another woman said, "Once they talk, they are too old to breastfeed," and someone else objected to breastfeeding a baby with teeth.

What I really wanted the class to understand is that when a mother breastfeeds an older child, she is nurturing the baby within that child. It is as if she is holding the tender baby that resides within the energetic body of her growing child. As time passes, the child matures, the baby disappears, and breastfeeding becomes a memory. Instead, I did my best to gather the class's attention and move on to another less controversial topic. Since then I have learned to stay away from the issue of extended breastfeeding unless specifically asked.

The emotional and physical benefits of breastfeeding do not diminish as your baby becomes a toddler or preschooler. Breastfeeding serves to lessen temper tantrums and helps a child to quickly fall asleep at naptime. Breastfeeding comforts a sick child and helps to speed recovery. The consistency of your breastfeeding relationship can serve as a stabilizing force within your child's life. I observed this firsthand when my son Max was four years old and needed to unexpectedly change preschools. When I explained to Max that he was going to a new bigger and busier preschool, he shrugged his shoulders and said, "That's okay as long as I can still have mama's." "Mama's" was our word for breastfeeding. Max continued breastfeeding and ended up loving his new preschool.

WILL BREASTFEEDING DAMAGE MY BABY'S TEETH?

It is well known that consuming formula, cow's milk, or fruit juice from a bottle just before bed or while sleeping can cause a child to develop severe tooth decay.[3] This occurs when formula, cow's milk, or juice drips from the bottle during the night and settles onto the surface of the teeth and provides a medium for the growth of cavity-causing plaque. Over time, the plaque proliferates and damages the integrity of the child's tooth enamel.[4] Preventing cavities and maintaining good dental health during childhood is critically important to the development of proper speech as well as normal dentition later in life.[5]

It is unlikely that breastfeeding during the night has the same potential to cause cavities in the way that bottle-feeding does. When compared with cow's milk, formula, and juice, breast milk does not have the same potential to cause tooth decay.[6] Furthermore, when breastfeeding, milk does not continually drip into a child's mouth and collect on the teeth the way it does with bottle-feeding. Breast milk alone is not likely to cause cavities, but the interaction of breast milk with food particles left on a child's teeth could lead to plaque and cavity formation. Therefore, to promote optimal dental health and prevent the formation of cavities, it is recommended that mothers remove plaque from their child's teeth with a toothbrush twice a day.[7]

HOW DO I EXPLAIN THAT WE ARE STILL BREASTFEEDING?

Sometimes extended breastfeeding creeps up on you. You might not have planned to breastfeed your baby into childhood, but now you cannot find a reason to stop. Although you and your child may be content to breastfeed into the future, you may find that your family and friends are uncomfortable with your breastfeeding relationship. That's what happened to my client Tori, who was breastfeeding her two-year-old daughter, Courtney. Tori and her husband were pleased that Courtney was a happy, healthy, breastfed child. However, when Tori's mother came to visit, she was shocked at the sight of Courtney breastfeeding. After Courtney went to bed, Tori's mother admonished Tori for allowing Courtney to continue breastfeeding "like a baby." Tori anticipated her mother's disapproval and responded by stating, "Breastfeeding before bedtime is part of the weaning process." This diffused the situation, and Tori and her mother agreed to disagree on the topic of breastfeeding Courtney.

HOW DO I STOP IF I AM READY?

All babies eventually stop breastfeeding on their own. Natural weaning is a process that occurs as your baby grows and matures. Baby-led weaning can have indistinct edges with lots of starts and stops before your baby bids a final farewell to breastfeeding. However, you may feel ready to stop breastfeeding before your baby does. If you have reached your breastfeeding goal, you can choose to play an active role in the weaning process. Use the following steps to make weaning a comfortable and positive experience for both of you.

Reduce your milk supply

If you have a full or nearly full milk supply, you will need to deliberately reduce your milk production as part of the weaning process. Suddenly stopping without lowering your milk supply may result in plugged ducts or mastitis. Safely reduce your supply by leaving your breasts comfortably full of milk. Breastfeed your baby, or pump enough to soften your breasts. In a short amount of time, your body will get the message to make less milk. Eventually, you will no longer feel the need to breastfeed or pump. The medication Sudafed can help to reduce your milk supply during the weaning process.[8]

Replace your breast milk

Your baby will need food and fluids in place of your breast milk. Cow's milk is not recommended for a baby under one year of age.[9] If your baby is younger than one, you will need to choose an appropriate formula to feed your baby. If your baby is eating solid food, plan to offer plenty of opportunities for your baby to eat at the times you would usually breastfeed.

Remain close

Weaning offers you the opportunity to enter into a new relationship with your baby. Replace the physical closeness of breastfeeding with new activities. Instead of breastfeeding, engage your older child in age-appropriate art projects, games, or cooking. When actively weaning an older child, avoid sitting on the sofa where you routinely breastfed. Offer your baby close physical contact by holding your baby in a backpack or baby carrier. Discover what you can do to help your baby or child move on to the next stage of your relationship.

SUMMARY OF BREASTFEEDING ABCs

Weaning is a process that begins when your baby is regularly consuming foods or drinks instead of breast milk. Ideally, this process occurs gradually over time. The best time to end your breastfeeding relationship is when both you and your baby are ready. It is normal and natural for your baby to breastfeed into toddlerhood or even early childhood. Breastfeeding continues to benefit your older baby physically and emotionally. All babies eventually stop breastfeeding on their own; however, if you reach your breastfeeding goal and feel ready to completely stop, you can accelerate the weaning process. To do this, you will need to reduce your milk supply and replace the breast milk in your baby's diet with age-appropriate nourishment.

A. AGE

Weaning begins with the regular introduction of solid food into your baby's daily diet. Most babies are ready to begin the experience of eating solid foods at around six months of age. Before six months of age, your breast milk provides your baby with optimal nutrition. Starting solids does not signal the end of breastfeeding. In fact, the AAP recommends that you continue to breastfeed until your baby's first birthday, and the WHO recommends continued breastfeeding for at least two years.

B. BABY-LED

When it comes to weaning, consider letting your baby lead the way. As your baby eats solid food and drinks from a cup, your breast milk still provides valuable nutrients and immune factors that are important to your baby's good health. Your breastfeeding relationship provides your baby with a secure safety net as your baby explores the world and tackles developmental milestones. All babies eventually completely wean, and your baby will let you know when the time is right to say good-bye to breastfeeding.

C. COMPLETE

Complete weaning does not occur suddenly. Weaning is a gradual process. If your baby suddenly refuses to breastfeed, it could be that your baby is having a nursing strike. This is your baby's way of telling you that something has upset his or her usual routine. Teething, illness, or hurried feedings are common causes of nursing strikes. Most of the time, nursing strikes are self-limiting and resolve within a day or two. Offering your baby a relaxed feeding during the night may help your baby to begin nursing again.

CHAPTER NINETEEN

First Baby Food:
Choosing Healthy Options

"I tried the powdered cereal myself,
and it tasted terrible."

—SUZANNE

Suzanne took five-month-old Dylan to the pediatrician's office for a check-up. After looking the baby over, the doctor told Suzanne that Dylan would soon be ready for solid food. Suzanne had been breastfeeding Dylan since birth and was excited about her baby starting solid foods. Although she couldn't wait to see how Dylan reacted to the taste of his first food, Suzanne was unsure how to integrate meals into her son's breastfeeding routine.

Once at home, Suzanne noticed that the first food listed on the printed feeding schedule from the doctor's office was rice cereal. Suzanne had planned to make homemade baby food out of apples, squash, and mashed bananas. She wondered if Dylan's first food had to be rice cereal as the doctor recommended. After reading the doctor's feeding schedule, Suzanne wasn't sure if her homemade baby food would be as good as the store-bought jars.

WHEN IS MY BABY READY FOR SOLID FOOD?

Suzanne's mother couldn't believe that Dylan had not yet tasted solid food. After all, she had mixed cereal into Suzanne's formula bottle when she was just weeks old. Although it is no longer recommended that infants be fed liquefied cereal from a baby bottle, experts still disagree as to when a breast-fed baby should be introduced to solid food. The AAP policy on breast-feeding recognizes that ideally all babies should have the benefit of mother's milk for the first six months of life.[1] However, the policy acknowledges the fact that each baby develops and matures at a unique pace. For instance, some babies may be ready for feeding experiences as early as four months old; others may not be ready until eight months of age.

It is important to realize that starting solid foods before six months of age does not increase a baby's caloric intake or provide a health advantage to your baby.[2] Delaying the introduction of solid foods for six months and continuing to breastfeed reduces the likelihood that your baby will contract a diarrheal illness.[3] Exclusive breastfeeding improves your baby's ability to crawl and walk by accelerating your baby's overall motor development.[4] Delaying solid foods benefits you as well. Exclusive breastfeeding for six months suppresses your fertility and acts as a natural form of birth control.[5] An additional benefit of prolonged breastfeeding is that it helps you lose weight and return to your pre-pregnancy size.[6]

When determining if your baby is ready for solid food, look for your baby's signs of feeding readiness. Not all babies are ready at exactly the same age. Some babies may be ready for meals before their peers, while other babies may need a little more time. All babies eventually learn to accept solid food. In order to eat, your baby should be able to sit in a high chair with an attached tray. To make eating possible, your baby's tongue thrust reflex should be fading. Tongue thrusting serves to protect your baby's throat and airway from foreign objects. This reflex will diminish as your baby becomes ready for the feeding experience. Finally, your baby should be aware and interested in whatever you and your family are eating. Your baby should seem hungry and literally grasp for the food that you eat.

WILL MY BREAST MILK PREPARE MY BABY FOR SOLID FOOD?

Like most mothers, Suzanne wanted Dylan to develop a lifelong love of healthy food. Without realizing it, Suzanne had begun influencing Dylan's food preferences well before he was born. Unbeknownst to her, the meals that Suzanne consumed while pregnant were reflected in the odor of the amniotic fluid that surrounded and protected Dylan in utero.[7] As he developed, Dylan was literally bathed in the scent and taste of his mother's daily diet. Following Dylan's birth, the foods Suzanne ate influenced both the scent and taste of her breast milk.

The shifting flavors of mother's milk serve as a form of sensory stimulation to a growing baby.[8] Daily variations of a mother's diet serve to stimulate a baby's appetite. This is particularly true when a mother eats a spicy meal. Mothers can easily influence their baby's future food preferences by consuming healthy nutritious foods during pregnancy and while breastfeeding. Before birth and by breastfeeding, a mother gives her baby the opportunity to experience the flavor of the foods he or she will one day eat in solid form.

DOES MY BABY NEED MANUFACTURED BABY FOOD?

Store-bought baby cereals were originally manufactured for bottle-fed babies who after a few months on formula needed extra iron and nutrients in their diet. The fact that the flavor of formula is always the same could potentially leave the bottle-fed baby starved for the sensory stimulation of other foods.[9] Regardless of how a baby is fed, over the years rice cereal has become synonymous with a baby's first solid food. Yet few breastfeeding mothers realize that their baby does not need store-bought cereal. Early introduction of these cereals could be a predisposing factor in the development of celiac disease.[10] In fact, feeling the need to limit exclusive breastfeeding to four months instead of six creates the impression that breastfed babies need specially manufactured foods or follow-up formulas.[11]

The reality is that your breast milk is more nutritious than commercial baby food. Up until the age of six months and possibly beyond, breastfeeding provides your baby with a perfect balance of easily digestible proteins, fats, and vitamins. The problem with beginning solids too early is that the food displaces a certain volume of nutrient-dense breast milk from your baby's daily diet. Feeding your baby early will not increase your baby's overall growth. The same holds true when it comes to your baby's iron levels. Babies born around their due dates are equipped with stores of iron and zinc that last until at least six months, at which time a baby can be introduced to iron-rich foods that are compatible with breastfeeding. Starting solids prior to six months has not been shown to affect iron levels, and administering iron drops to babies who have adequate iron stores of their own does not improve the baby's overall growth and may actually limit growth.[12]

SHOULD I SPOON-FEED MY BABY?

Babies instinctively prefer the milk of their mothers. This is true when it comes to solid food as well. The bland taste and pasty texture of traditional baby cereal does not make an appealing first food. When offered cereal, babies clearly prefer it mixed with their mother's breast milk as opposed to cereal mixed with plain water.[13] Babies appreciate the flavors of natural foods just as adults do. Luckily for babies, the world is full of a variety of whole foods that when appropriately prepared make delicious first foods.

One of the advantages of breastfeeding is that your baby cannot overfeed. Your baby will signal satiety by simply ending a feeding. The proteins and hormones in your milk help your baby to regulate caloric intake. During a feeding, your baby takes the amount of breast milk that is appropriate for his or her stomach size; in this way, breastfeeding plays a role in preventing future obesity.[14] The same principle applies when introducing your breastfed baby to solid food.

Spoon-feeding your baby may lead your baby to take more than he or she is ready for. Letting your baby pick up soft pieces of food and self-feed prevents overeating. Providing your baby with the opportunity to touch, hold, and self-feed enables your baby to control the pace of eating. This leads to a positive feeding experience. Whether you spoon-feed or let your baby self-feed, it is going to be an equally messy meal!

WHAT ARE SELF-FEEDING FOODS?

When Dylan was six months old, he began to grasp and hold objects in his hands and would put almost anything in his mouth. It seemed natural for Suzanne to take advantage of Dylan's developmental interest by providing the opportunity for Dylan to feed himself. Suzanne chose carrots for Dylan's first food, a vegetable she frequently ate herself. She peeled and steamed the carrots until they were very soft. After breastfeeding Dylan, Suzanne sat him in his high chair and put the cooled carrots on his tray. To pique Dylan's interest and to let him know that carrots were meant for eating, she pureed some of the cooked carrots and offered them to Dylan with her finger. Without any further coaxing, Dylan took over and did his best to feed himself the carrots.

The first foods you choose for your baby should complement your breastfeeding relationship, not replace it. Select foods for your baby that are part of your regular diet. Keep in mind that the flavor of your breast milk is influenced by the foods that you eat. Your baby may be more willing to try a familiar food as opposed to one that you never eat. As your baby adapts to eating solid foods, regular meals will take the place of a certain volume of your breast milk. Your breast milk should be replaced only with protein and vitamin-rich solid foods. Babies don't need foods with added butter, sugar, or salt.

HOW DO I PREPARE FOOD FOR MY BABY?

Store-bought powdered cereal does not have to be your baby's first food. However, if you prefer to start your baby with cereal, mixing it with your breast milk will make it more palatable. Otherwise, select foods that you frequently eat. Foods that you and your family enjoy will complement your breastfeeding relationship. Breastfeed your baby before offering a solid meal. If your baby is ready for the experience of eating solid food, he or she will show interest in eating after breastfeeding. Use a fork, blender, food processor, or baby food grinder to puree or soften cooked or very ripe foods. For advice on preparing and introducing healthy baby food, consult the book *Whole Foods for the Whole Family* published by the La Leche League and *Whole Foods for Babies and Toddlers* by Margaret Kenda.

When shopping for commercially prepared baby food, choose jars that contain a single food rather than combined foods. Feeding your baby one type of food at a time allows you to gauge your baby's reaction and tolerance to the food. Since food allergies tend to run in families, avoid exposing your baby to foods to which you are allergic. Hold off on highly allergic foods like nuts, peanuts, and shellfish until your baby is over one-year-old.

Fruits and vegetables

Ripe bananas make an ideal first food for your baby. Introduce your baby to mashed or pureed bananas on your finger or with a spoon. Next, provide your baby the opportunity to pick up pieces of banana and self-feed. Ripe avocados also make excellent baby food. Be sure the avocado is soft enough to be mashed between your baby's gums. Other whole foods include cooked carrots, potatoes, squash, and peaches. Homemade baby food can be frozen in ice cube trays, and the frozen cubes can be stored in freezer bags to use later.

Protein

Breast milk serves as the primary source of protein for your baby's first year of life. If you and your family eat meat, your baby can have it in pureed form. Animal meat is a good source of protein, iron, and zinc. Vegetarian babies can be introduced to tofu and cooked beans as a protein source. Yogurt and other foods containing cow's milk protein can be gradually offered as your baby approaches one year of age.

Grains

Grains include cooked pasta, rice, and toast that older babies can gum or chew. Your baby will enjoy picking up and self-feeding individual pieces of dry cereal. Cheerios are ideal for this developmental task because they easily dissolve in your baby's mouth. Continuing to breastfeed may be especially important when introducing your baby to foods that contain gluten. Gluten is a wheat protein found in breads and cereal products. The inability to digest gluten is called celiac disease. The only treatment for celiac disease is to completely abstain from products that contain gluten. Being breastfed during the period of introduction to foods containing gluten has a protective effect against the development of celiac disease.[15]

DO I NEED TO INTRODUCE SOLIDS IN A SPECIFIC ORDER?

Nearly all of my clients receive painfully detailed feeding directions from their pediatrician's office. The instructions spell out in excruciating detail the measured amount and exact order in which each fruit or vegetable is to be spoon-fed to their baby. Usually rice cereal tops the list. This mother-led feeding style does not complement a breastfeeding relationship.

For the breastfeeding couple, the experience of eating solid food should mirror their breastfeeding relationship. A mother can entice her baby by offering a ripe fruit or vegetable that is part of her diet and readily available. Just as with breastfeeding, babies will regulate their intake of whole foods. Because solid food will displace some of the high-quality protein and nutrients that breast milk provides your baby, the La Leche League recommends breastfeeding babies be offered protein-containing foods early in their feeding experience.[16] Examples of high-protein foods are meat, tofu, and cooked black beans. As opposed to spoon-feeding powdered cereal, you can offer cooked pasta and whole grain bread in a form that your baby can pick up. This way, your baby can control the pace of the meal. Cow's milk and dairy foods can be offered when your baby is closer to one year old.

As your baby consumes more solid food and naturally breastfeeds less often, your milk supply will adjust accordingly. During this time of transition, your baby may make up for this reduction in breastfeeding by waking up more often during the night to breastfeed. This increase in nighttime feeding is temporary and will end as your baby integrates solid foods with breastfeeding. Like all developmental feats, learning to eat solid foods can be an unpredictable process. Your baby may thoroughly enjoy eating cooked carrots one day only to refuse them the next. This finicky behavior is normal. During the process of adapting to solid meals, your baby's appetite may wax and wane. If your baby seems uninterested in eating or refuses food altogether, simply try again later. Breast milk is still your baby's main source of nutrients during this transition to solid meals.

Babies adapt to food at their own pace. Your baby may readily eat several solid meals a day, or your baby may accept no more than a taste. Trust your baby to instinctively know when he or she is ready to eat. More than one of my clients shared her feelings of frustration after watching an elaborate assortment of artfully arranged baby food go to waste because her baby was uninterested in eating that day. Some day your child will appreciate your culinary efforts. Until then, offer your baby simply prepared nutritious foods at appropriate intervals. Just as with breastfeeding, your baby will eat when the time is right.

HOW WILL I KNOW IF MY BABY HAS A FOOD ALLERGY?

I can't remember how old my son Max was when I gave him a teething biscuit to hold in his hands. It was a summer afternoon, and he was reclining in his baby seat, which I had placed on the kitchen table beneath the ceiling fan. Like I said, I don't remember exactly how old he was, but I remember exactly what happened when he brought the innocent-looking biscuit to his lips. Within an instant, his skin turned scarlet, and a colony of hives sprung up across his face. Up until that moment, I had no reason to suspect that Max harbored a food allergy. A visit to the allergist confirmed that Max was severely allergic to cow's milk protein, an ingredient in that awful biscuit.

From then on, I carried an EpiPen everywhere we went. I purged the house of cow's milk and dairy-containing foods. I obsessively read and reread food labels for evidence of hidden allergens. All food appeared suspicious and threatening. Even the tiniest crumb that crossed our path took on the sinister aura of a concealed allergen. For the next year, mealtime became a great source of anxiety for me.

Oddly enough, it was by mistake—my mistake—that I discovered Max had overcome his allergy. While sitting together at the table, I handed Max a cup meant for his sister. The cup contained leftover vanilla milkshake from a restaurant. After recognizing my mistake, I ran for the EpiPen. I waited and expected the worst. Nothing happened. No hives, no swelling, no scarlet skin. The allergist later proclaimed that Max was healed of his allergy and slowly we reintroduced dairy into Max's diet. Eventually, I stopped carrying the EpiPen.

A sudden allergic reaction to food like anaphylaxis and hives is impossible to miss and likely to occur immediately after consuming a food item. The most common foods that cause allergy are cow's milk, eggs, soy, peanuts, tree nuts, wheat, fish, and shellfish.[17] Merely touching the allergen can be enough to cause symptoms in some children. While an allergy is not subtle, some food intolerances can be harder to recognize because they can occur twenty-four to seventy-two hours after eating the offending food.[18] Symptoms can include dermatitis, reflux, and diarrhea.[19]

If your child has a food allergy or intolerance, whether the reaction is immediate or delayed, eliminate the food from your child's diet. It may be possible to test your child to identify a food allergy. Consult a pediatric allergist to see if skin testing is appropriate for your child's situation. This is especially important if food allergies run in your family. Thankfully, many children outgrow a food allergy or intolerance by the time they are ready for school.

SUMMARY OF BREASTFEEDING ABCs

Breast milk provides your baby with the perfect balance of nutrients for the first six months of your baby's life. Waiting until your baby is six months old before introducing solid foods benefits you as well as your baby. Babies who are exclusively breastfed for six months have lower rates of illness and better motor development than babies who are fed solid foods before six months of age. Exclusive breastfeeding helps you to lose weight and serves as natural birth control by delaying the return of your fertility. Babies mature and develop at different rates. When your baby is ready for solid food, he or she will seem hungry and begin to reach for food. Breastfed babies do not need processed rice cereal. Allow your baby the opportunity to self-feed. Begin with ripe bananas, avocados, and cooked vegetables. Foods should be nutritious and complement your breastfeeding relationship rather than replace it.

A. APPETITE

Babies differ in their developmental readiness for solid foods. Some babies may be ready as early as four months while other babies may not be ready until the age of eight months. In general, your breast milk provides all the nutrients your baby needs for the first six months of life and probably longer. Observe your baby for signs of feeding readiness. First, your baby

should be able to sit in a high chair. Next, your baby's tongue thrust reflex should diminish. Finally, your baby will develop an appetite and begin reaching for solid foods. When you eat, your baby will seem hungry
and grasp for your food. It is normal for your baby's appetite to vary from
one day to the next. A food that was your baby's favorite one day may go
to waste the following day. An unpredictable, finicky appetite is a normal
part of the process of learning to eat.

B. BABY FOOD

Ideally, your baby's solid food should mirror your breast milk. The foods
that you eat on a daily basis are reflected in the flavor of your breast milk.
When selecting solid food for your baby, let your own diet guide you. The
foods that you eat will be familiar to your baby and will therefore be easier for your baby to accept. It is not necessary to purchase commercial
baby food in jars unless you want to; otherwise, select whole foods that
are readily available. When preparing your baby's food, you do not need
extra butter, salt, or sugar. Babies appreciate the flavors of natural foods.

C. CEREAL

It has become a popular practice to offer processed rice cereal as a baby's first
food; however, breastfeeding babies do not need this manufactured product. Simply put, the lackluster flavor of powdered cereal does not make for
a palatable first food. In fact, babies tend to prefer the flavors of real food.
Although most prescribed feeding plans begin with powdered cereal, the
early introduction of these cereals will not improve your baby's overall
growth and may, in fact, contribute to the development of celiac disease in
susceptible babies. Rather than reconstituting and spoon-feeding your baby
powdered cereals early on, wait to introduce grains when your baby is able
to self-feed cooked pasta, toast, and Cheerios.

Notes

Chapter 1. Thinking with a Breastfeeding Mindset

1. B. Heiser and M. Walker, "Selling out Mothers and Babies, Marketing of Breast Milk Substitutes in the USA," (2007): available from marsha@naba-breastfeeding.org.

2. Massachusetts Breastfeeding Coalition, "What's Wrong with Those Cute Formula 'Gift' Bags?" (2006): www.massbfc.org.

3. J. Kulski and P. Hartmann, "Changes in Human Milk Composition During the Initiation of Lactation," *The Australian Journal of Experimental Biology and Medical Science* 59 (1981): 101–114.

4. W. Diehl-Jones and D. Askin, "Nutritional Modulation of Neonatal Outcomes," *AACN Clinical Issues Advanced Practice Acute Critical Care* 15 (2004): 83–96.

5. M. Walker, "Just One Bottle Won't Hurt"—Or Will It?" *Supplementation of the Breastfed Baby* (2007): www.massbfc.org/formula/bottle.html.

6. L. Mitoulas et al., "Variation in Fat, Lactose, and Protein in Human Milk Over 24 Hours and Throughout the First Year of Lactation," *British Journal of Nutrition* 88 (2002): 29–37.

7. E. Mortensen, "The Association Between Duration of Breastfeeding and Adult Intelligence," *JAMA* 287 (2002): 2365–2371.

8. J. Riordan, *Breastfeeding and Human Lactation,* 3rd ed. (Sudbury, MA: Jones and Bartlett Publishers, 2005), 367–369.

9. W. Diehl-Jones and D. Askin, "Nutritional Modulation of Neonatal Out-comes," *AACN Clinical Issues Advanced Practice Acute Critical Care* 15 (2004): 83-96.

10. P. Hartmann, "Initiation of Lactation in Term and Pre-Term Mothers," Lec-ture at 10th Annual Breastfeeding Conference; Baystate Health Systems Office of Continuing Education (2005).

11. J. Mennella, "Mother's Milk: A Medium for Early Flavor Experiences," *Journal of Human Lactation* 11 (1995): 39–45.

12. S. Daly and P. Hartmann, "Infant Demand and Milk Supply. Part 2: The Short-Term Control of Milk Synthesis in Lactating Women," *Journal of Human Lactation* 11 (1995): 27–37.

Chapter 2. Finding a Breastfeeding-Friendly Doctor

1. J. Fulhan et al., "Update on Pediatric Nutrition: Breastfeeding, Infant Nutrition, and Growth," *Current Opinion in Pediatrics* 15 (2003): 323–332.

2. AAP Policy Statement, "Breastfeeding and the Use of Human Milk," *Pediatrics* 115 (2005): 496–506.

3. M. Pessl, "Exclusive Breastfeeding: Does It Matter?" *Connecticut Breastfeeding Coalition Lecture Syllabus* (2006): 1–8.

4. J. Winberg, "Mother and Newborn Baby: Mutual Regulation of Physiology and Behavior—A Selective Review," *Developmental Psychobiology* 47 (2005): 217–229; K. Dewey, "What Is the Optimal Age for Introduction of Complimentary Foods?" *Nestle Nutrition Workshop Series* 58 (2006): 161–170.

5. M. Sowers et al., "Changes in Bone Density with Lactation," *JAMA* 296 (1993): 3130–3135.

6. T. Hale, *Medications and Mothers' Milk,* 12th ed. (Amarillo, TX: Hale Publishing, 2006), 196–197.

7. Ibid, 350–353.

8. Ibid, 426–427.

9. J. Panksepp, "Oxytocin Effects on Emotional Processes: Separation Distress, Social Bonding, and Relationships to Psychiatric Disorders," *Annals of the New York Academy of Sciences* 652 (1992): 243–252.

Chapter 3. Planning for a Gentle Birth

1. Y. Beilin et al., "Effect of Labor Epidural Analgesia With and Without Fentanyl on Infant Breastfeeding," *Anesthesiology* 103 (2005): 1211–1217.

2. M. Walker, "Do Labor Medications Affect Breastfeeding?" *Journal of Human Lactation* 13 (1997): 131–137.

3. Ibid.

4. A. Ransjo-Arvidson et al., "Maternal Analgesia During Labor Disturbs Newborn Behavior: Effects on Breastfeeding, Temperature, and Crying," *Birth* 28 (2001): 5–12.

5. J. Riordan et al., "The Effect of Labor Pain Relief Medication on Neonatal Suckling and Breastfeeding Duration," *Journal of Human Lactation* 16 (2000): 7–12.

6. A. Ransjo-Arvidson et al., 5–12.

7. K. Dewey et al., "Risk Factors for Sub-Optimal Infant Breastfeeding Behavior, Delayed Onset of Lactation, and Excess Neonatal Weight Loss," *Pediatrics* 112 (2003): 607–619.

8. Ibid.

9. P. England and R. Horowitz, *Birthing from Within* (Albuquerque: Partera Press, 1998), 207–212.

10. K. Scheer and J. Nubar, "Variation of Fetal Presentation with Gestational Age," *American Journal of Obstetrics and Gynecology* 125 (1976): 269.

11. A. Vidaeff, "Breech Delivery Before and After the Term Breech Trial," *Clinical Obstetrics* 49 (2006): 198–210.

Chapter 4. How to Hold Your Baby After Birth

1. J. Winberg, "Mother and Newborn Baby: Mutual Regulation of Physiology and Behavior—A Selective Review," *Developmental Psychobiology* 47 (2005): 217–219.

2. Ibid.

3. N. Bergman, "Skin-to-Skin Contact, Breastfeeding, and Perinatal Neuroscience," Hollister Breastfeeding Program (2006): 1–67; www.kangaroomothercare.com.

4. AAP Policy Statement, "Breastfeeding and the Use of Human Milk," *Pediatrics* 115 (2005): 496–506.

Chapter 5. Avoiding Separation After Birth

1. S. Ludington-Hoe et al., "Infant Crying: Nature, Physiologic Consequences, and Select Intervention," *Neonatal Network* 21 (2002): 29–36.

2. Ibid.

3. Ibid.

4. L. Gray et al., "Breastfeeding Is Analgesic in Healthy Newborns," *Pediatrics* 109 (2002): 590–593.

5. J. Winberg, "Mother and Newborn Baby: Mutual Regulation of Physiology and Behavior—A Selective Review," *Developmental Psychobiology* 47 (2005), 217–229.

6. L. Gray et al., 590–593.

7. Ibid.

8. M. Keefe, "The Impact of Infant Rooming-In on Maternal Sleep at Night," *JOGNN* 17 (1988): 122–126.

9. M. Freeman et al., "Prolactin: Structure, Function, and Regulation of Secretion," *Physiological Reviews* 80 (2000): 1523–1631.

10. J. Winberg, "Mother and Newborn Baby: Mutual Regulation of Physiology and Behavior—A Selective Review," *Developmental Psychobiology* 47 (2005): 217–229.

Chapter 6. Bottle and Breast: Preventing Feeding Confusion

1. M. Neifert et al., "Nipple Confusion: Toward a Formal Definition," *The Journal of Pediatrics* 126 (1995), 125–129.

2. M. Benis, "Are Pacifiers Associated with Early Weaning from Breastfeeding?" *Advances in Neonatal Care* 2 (2002): 259–266.

3. K. Hoover, "The Link Between Infants' Oral Thrush and Nipple and Breast Pain in Lactating Women" (Mortan, PA: Self-Published Handout, 2001), 1–4.

4. K. Dewey et al., "Risk Factors for Sub-Optimal Infant Breastfeeding Behavior, Delayed Onset of Lactation, and Excess Neonatal Weight Loss," *Pediatrics* 112 (2003): 607–619.

5. S. Ludington-Hoe et al., "Infant Crying: Nature, Physiologic Consequences, and Select Interventions," *Neonatal Network* 21 (2002): 29–36.

6. M. Walker, "Just One Bottle Won't Hurt"—Or Will It?" *Supplementation of the Breastfed Baby* (2007): www.massbfc.org/formula/bottle.html.

7. Ibid.

8. J. Morrill et al., "Risk Factors for Mammary Candidiasis Among Lactating Women," *JOGNN* 34 (2005): 37–45.

9. J. Willumsen et al., "Breastmilk RNA Viral Load in HIV-Infected South African Women: Effects of Subclinical Mastitis and Infant Feeding," *AIDS* 17 (2003): 407–414.

10. AAP Policy Statement, "Breastfeeding and the Use of Human Milk," *Pediatrics* 115 (2005): 496–506.

11. K. Dewey et al., 607–619.

12. G. Souto et al., "The Impact of Breast Reduction Surgery on Breastfeeding Performance," *Journal of Human Lactation* 19 (2003): 43–49.

Chapter 7. The Signals That Will Let You Know When to Feed Your Baby

1. S. Daly and P. Hartmann, "Infant Demand and Milk Supply. Part 2: The Short-Term Control of Milk Synthesis in Lactating Women," *Journal of Human Lactation* 11 (1995): 27–37.

2. Ibid.

3. M. Walker, *Core Curriculum for Lactation Consultant Practice* (Sudbury, MA: Jones and Bartlett Publishers, 2002), 47–60.

4. S. Daly et al., "Degree of Breast Emptying Explains Changes in the Fat Content, But Not Fatty Acid Composition of Human Milk," *Experimental Physiology* 78 (1993): 741–755.

Chapter 8. Getting Comfortable
1. S. Daly and P. Hartmann, "Infant Demand and Milk Supply. Part 2: The Short-Term Control of Milk Synthesis in Lactating Women," *Journal of Human Lactation* 11 (1995): 27–37.

Chapter 9. How to Avoid Becoming Overwhelmed
1. J. Winberg, "Mother and Newborn Baby: Mutual Regulation of Physiology and Behavior—A Selective Review," *Developmental Psychobiology* 47 (2005): 217–229.

2. K. Kendall-Tackett, "Post-Partum Depression and the Breastfeeding Mother, Part I: Cause and Consequences," *La Leche League International Independent Study Module* 5 (2003): 1–31.

3. V. Whiffen and I. Gotlib, "Infants of Post-Partum Depressed Mothers; Temperament and Cognitive Status," *Journal of Abnormal Psychology* 98 (1989): 274–279.

4. E. Mezzacappa and E. Katkin, "Breastfeeding Is Associated with Reduced Perceived Stress and Negative Mood in Mothers," *Health Psychology* 21 (2002): 187–193.

5. AAP Policy Statement, "Breastfeeding and the Use of Human Milk," *Pediatrics* 115 (2005): 496–506.

6. Ibid.

Chapter 10. How to Build a Strong Supply of Mature Milk
1. J. Riordan, *Breastfeeding and Human Lactation*, 3rd ed. (Sudbury, MA: Jones and Bartlett Publishers, 2005), 97–99.

2. M. Freeman et al., "Prolactin: Structure, Function, and Regulation of Secretion," *Physiological Reviews* 80 (2000): 8–31.

3. J. Riordan, 73–80.

4. Ibid.

5. G. Souto et al., "The Impact of Breast Reduction Surgery on Breastfeeding Performance," *Journal of Human Lactation* 19 (2003): 43–49.

6. K. Dewey et al., "Risk Factors for Sub-Optimal Infant Breastfeeding Behavior, Delayed Onset of Lactation, and Excess Neonatal Weight Loss," *Pediatrics* 112 (2003): 607–619.

7. Ibid.

8. Ibid.

9. Ibid.

10. K. Kennedy, "Premature Introduction of Progestin-Only Contraceptive Methods During Lactation," *Contraception* 55 (1997): 347–350.

Chapter 11. How to Know When Pain Is a Problem

1. J. Fulhan et al., "Update on Pediatric Nutrition: Breastfeeding, Infant Nutrition, and Growth." *Current Opinion in Pediatrics* 15 (2003): 323–332; J. Anderson et al., "Breast-feeding and Cognitive Development: A Meta-Analysis." *American Journal of Clinical Nutrition* 70 (1999): 525–535.

2. K. Tanguay et al., "Nipple Candidiasis Among Breastfeeding Mothers," *Canadian Family Physician* 40 (1994): 1407–1413.

3. M. Walker, "Mastitis in Lactating Woman," *La Leche League International Independent Study Module* 6 (2004): 1–19.

4. Ibid.

5. J. Riordan, *Breastfeeding and Human Lactation,* 3rd ed. (Sudbury, MA: Jones and Bartlett Publishers, 2005), 252–253.

6. K. Tanguay et al., 1407–1413.

7. J. Morrill et al., "Risk Factors for Mammary Candidiasis Among Lactating Women," *JOGNN* 34 (2005): 37–45.

8. K. Hoover, *The Link Between Infants' Oral Thrush and Nipple and Breast Pain in Lactating Women*, 4th ed. (Mortan, PA: Self-Published Handout, 2001), 1–4.

9. S. Graves et al., "Painful Nipples in Nursing Mothers: Fungal or Staphylococcal?" *Australian Family Physician* 32 (2003): 570–571.

10. K. Hoover, 1–4.

11. T. Hale, *Medications and Mothers' Milk*, 12th ed. (Amarillo, TX: Hale Publishing, 2006), 350–354.

12. Ibid, 403.

13. J. Ballard et al., "Ankyloglossia: Assessment, Incidence, and Effect of Frenuloplasty on the Breastfeeding Dyad," *Pediatrics* 110 (November 2002): 1–6.

14. Ibid.

Chapter 12. How to Maintain a Strong Supply of Milk

1. M. Cregan et al., "Milk Prolactin, Feed Volume, and Duration Between Feeds in Women Breastfeeding Their Full-Term Infants Over a 24-hour Period," *Experimental Physiology* 87 (2002): 207–214.

2. S. Daly et al., "Degree of Breast Emptying Explains Changes in the Fat Content, But Not Fatty Acid Composition, of Human Milk," *Experimental Physiology* 78 (1993): 741–755.

3. D. Cox et al., "Blood and Milk Prolactin and the Rate of Milk Synthesis in Women," *Experimental Physiology* 81 (1996): 1007–1020.

4. M. Cregan et al., 207–214.

5. J. Riordan, *Breastfeeding and Human Lactation*, 3rd ed. (Sudbury, MA: Jones and Bartlett Publishers, 2005), 119–120.

6. J. Fulhan et al., "Update on Pediatric Nutrition: Breastfeeding, Infant Nutrition, and Growth," *Current Opinion in Pediatrics* 15 (2003): 223–232.

7. T. Hale, *Medications and Mothers' Milk* (Amarillo, TX: Hale Publishing, 2006), 343–344.

8. Ibid, 277–278.

9. Ibid, 591–593.

10. Ibid, 749–750.

11. S. Daly and P. Hartmann, "Infant Demand and Milk Supply. Part 2: The Short-Term Control of Milk Synthesis in Lactating Woman," *Journal of Human Lactation* 11 (1995): 27–37.

Chapter 13. How Do I Do This in Public?

1. E. Baldwin and K. Friedman, "A Current Summary of Breastfeeding Legislation in the U.S.," La Leche League International, 2006, www.llli.org/Law/Bills6.html.

2. Connecticut General Statute-2007, "A Current Summary of Breastfeeding Legislation: Summary of Enacted Breastfeeding Legislation," http://www.lalecheleague.org/Law/Bills12.html.

3. CDC Breastfeeding National Immunization Data, "Breastfeeding Practices: Results from the 2003 National Immunization Survey," http://www.cdc.gov/breastfeeding/NIS_data/index.htm.

4. J. Hyams et al., "Effect of Infant Formula on Stool Characteristics of Young Infants," *Pediatrics* 95 (1995): 50–54.

Chapter 14. Can I Eat My Favorite Foods?

1. J. Mennella and G. Beauchamp, "Maternal Diet Alters the Sensory Qualities of Human Milk and the Nursling's Behavior," *Pediatrics* 88 (1991): 737–744.

2. J. Winberg, "Mother and Newborn Baby: Mutual Regulation of Physiology and Behavior—A Selective Review," *Developmental Psychobiology* 47 (2005): 217–229.

3. J. Roepke, "Appropriate Introduction of Complementary Foods into the Diet of the Exclusively Breastfed Infant," *La Leche League International Study Module* 14 (2005): 1–16.

4. I. Jakobsson, "Food Antigens in Human Milk," *European Journal of Clinical Nutrition* 45 (1991): 29–33.

5. T. Hale, *Medications and Mothers' Milk*, 12th ed. (Amarillo, TX: Hale Publishing, 2006), 121–123.

6. Ibid, 322–323.

7. Food and Drug Administration, "Backgrounder for the 2004 FDA/EPA Consumer Advisory: What You Need to Know About Mercury in Fish and Shellfish," http://www.fda.gov/oc/opacom/hottopics/mercury/backgrounder.html.

8. Ibid.

9. I. Griffin and S. Abrams, "Iron Metabolism in Human Milk–Fed Infants," *La Leche League International Study Module* 11 (2003): 4–19.

10. Ibid.

11. Ibid, 18.

12. A. Mangels and V. Messina, "Considerations in Planning Vegan Diets: Infants," *Journal of the American Dietetic Association* 101 (2001): 670–677.

13. M. J. Heinig, "Vitamin D and the Breastfed Infant: Controversies and Concerns," *Journal of Human Lactation* 19 (2003): 247–249.

14. AAP Policy Statement, "Breastfeeding and the Use of Human Milk," *Pediatrics* 115 (2005): 496–506.

15. K. Allen et al., "Food Allergy in Childhood," *MJA* 185 (2006): 394–400.

16. Ibid.

17. Ibid.

Chapter 15. Yes, You *Can* Get Some Sleep

1. S. Rivkees, "Developing Circadian Rhythmicity in Infants," *Pediatrics* 112 (2003): 373–381.

2. M. Cregan et al., "Milk Prolactin, Feed Volume, and Duration Between Feeds in Women Breastfeeding Their Full-Term Infants Over a 24-Hour Period," *Experimental Physiology* 87 (2002): 207–214.

3. S. Rivkees, 373–381.

4. S. Quillin and L. Glenn, "Interaction Between Feeding Method and Co-Sleeping on Maternal/Newborn Sleep," *JOGNN* 33 (2004): 580–588.

5. Ibid.

6. National Sleep Foundation, "2002 Sleep in America Poll," http://www.sleep foundation.org.

Chapter 16. How to Make Breastfeeding Compatible with Family Life

1. T. Lavender et al., "Breastfeeding and Family Life," *Natural and Child Nutrition* (2006): 145–155; V. Swanson and K. G. Power, "Initiation and Continuation

of Breastfeeding: Theory of Planned Behavior," *Journal of Advanced Nursing* 50 (2004): 272–282.

2. J. Riordan, *Breastfeeding and Human Lactation,* 3rd ed. (Sudbury, MA: Jones and Bartlett Publishers, 2005), 634–635.

3. M. Labbok et al., "Multicenter Study of the Lactational Amenorrhea Method (LAM): I. Efficacy, Duration, and Implications for Clinical Application," *Contraception* 55 (1997): 327–336.

4. S. T. Truitt et al., "Combined Hormonal Versus Nonhormonal Versus Progestin Only Contraception in Lactation," *The Cochrane Collaboration* 1 (2007): 1–14.

5. J. T. Queenan, "Contraception and Breastfeeding," *Clinical Obstetrics and Gynecology* 47 (2004): 734–739.

Chapter 17. Combining Breastfeeding with Your Career

1. L. Lewallen et al., "Breastfeeding Support and Early Cessation," *JOGNN* 35 (2006): 166–172.

2. Connecticut General Statute-1997, "A Current Summary of Breastfeeding Legislation in the U.S.," www.lalecheleague.org/Law/Bills12.html.

3. M. Zinaman et al., "Acute Prolactin and Oxytocin Responses and Milk Yield to Infant Suckling and Artificial Methods of Expression in Lactating Women," *Pediatrics* 89 (1992): 437–440.

Chapter 18. When Is the Right Time to Wean?

1. AAP Policy Statement, "Breastfeeding and the Use of Human Milk," *Pediatrics* 115 (2005): 496–506.

2. Ibid.

3. N. Ersin et al., "Association of Maternal-Child Characteristics as a Factor in Early Childhood Caries Salivary Bacterial Counts," *Journal of Dentistry for Children* 73 (2006): 105–111.

4. K. Marinelli, "Breastfeeding and Oral Health: Early Childhood Caries," Lecture Syllabus—3rd Annual Conference Breastfeeding for Health Team Member 2003 (Chicago, IL), 1–7.

5. Ibid.

6. AAPD Policy Statement, "Policy on Dietary Recommendations for Infants, Children, and Adolescents," *Pediatric Dentistry* 27 (2005–2006): 36–37.

7. N. Ersin et al., 105–111.

8. T. Hale, *Medications and Mothers' Milk*, 12th ed. (Amarillo, TX: Hale Publishing, 2006), 749–750.

9. AAP Policy Statement, "Breastfeeding and the Use of Human Milk," *Pediatrics* 115 (2005): 496–506.

Chapter 19. First Baby Food: Choosing Healthy Options

1. AAP Policy Statement, "Breastfeeding and the Use of Human Milk," *Pediatrics* 115 (2005): 496–506.

2. K. Dewey, "What Is the Optimal Age for Introduction of Complementary Foods?" Nestle Nutrition Workshop Series 58 (2006): 161–170.

3. Ibid.

4. Ibid.

5. M. Labbok, et al., "Multicenter Study of the Lactational Amenhorrea Method (LAM): I. Efficacy, Duration, and Complications for Clinical Application," *Contraception* 55 (1997): 327–336.

6. K. Dewey, 161–170.

7. J. Mennella et al., "Garlic Ingestion by Pregnant Women Alters the Odor of Amniotic Fluid," *Chemical Senses* 20 (1995): 207–209.

8. J. Mennella, "Mother's Milk: A Medium for Early Flavor Experiences," *Journal of Human Lactation* 11 (1995): 39–45.

9. Ibid.

10. A. Akobeng et al., "Effect of Breast Feeding on Risk of Coeliac Disease: A Systematic Review and Meta-Analysis of Observational Studies," *Archives of Disease in Childhood* 91 (2006): 39–43.

11. H. Borresen, "Rethinking Current Recommendations to Introduce Solid Foods Between Four and Six Months to Exclusively Breastfeeding Infants," *Journal of Human Lactation* 11 (1995): 201–204.

12. I. Griffin and S. Abrams, "Iron Metabolism in Human Milk–Fed Infants," La Leche League International Independent Study Module 11 (2003): 2–19.

13. J. Mennella and G. Beauchamp, "Mothers' Milk Enhances the Acceptance of Cereal During Weaning," *Pediatric Research* 41 (1997): 188–192.

14. AAP Policy Statement, "Prevention of Pediatric Overweight and Obesity," *Pediatrics* 112 (2003): 424–430.

15. A. Akobeng et al., 39–43.

16. J. Roepke, "Appropriate Introduction of Complementary Foods into the Diet of the Exclusively Breastfed Infant," La Leche League International Independent Study Module 14 (2005): 1–12.

17. K. Allen et al., "Food Allergy in Childhood," *MJA Practice Essentials* 185 (2006): 394–400.

18. Ibid.

19. Ibid.

Bibliography

AAP Policy Statement. "Breastfeeding and the Use of Human Milk." *Pediatrics* 115 (2005): 496–506.

Akobeng, A., et al. "Effect of Breast Feeding on Risk of Coeliac Disease: A Systematic Review and Meta-Analysis of Observational Studies." *Archives of Disease in Childhood* 91 (2006): 39–43.

Allen, K., et al. "Food Allergy in Childhood." *MJA* 185 (2006): 394–400.

Anderson, J., et al. "Breastfeeding and Cognitive Development: Meta-Analysis." *American Journal of Clinical Nutrition* 70 (1999): 525–535.

Baldwin, E., and K. Friedman. "A Current Summary of Breastfeeding Legislation in the U.S." La Leche League International website, 2006.

Ballard, J., et al. "Ankyloglossia: Assessment, Incidence, and Effect of Frenuloplasty on the Breastfeeding Dyad." *Pediatrics* 110 (November 2002): 1–6.

Beilin, Y., et al. "Effect of Labor Epidural Analgesia with and without Fentanyl on Infant Breastfeeding." *Anesthesiology* 103 (2005): 1211–1217.

Benis, M. "Are Pacifiers Associated with Early Weaning from Breastfeeding?" *Advances in Neonatal Care* 2 (2002): 259–266.

Bergmann, N. "Skin-to-Skin Contact, Breastfeeding, and Perinatal Neuroscience." Hollister Breastfeeding Program 2006, 1–67; www.kangaroomothercare.com.

Borresen, H. "Rethinking Current Recommendations to Introduce Solid Foods Between Four and Six Months to Exclusively Breastfeeding Infants." *Journal of Human Lactation* 11 (1995): 201–204.

Connecticut General Statute-1997. "A Current Summary of Breastfeeding Legislation in the U.S."; www.lalecheleague.org/Law/Bills12.html.

Cox, D., et al. "Blood and Milk Prolactin and the Rate of Milk Synthesis in Women." *Experimental Physiology* 81 (1996): 1007–1020.

Cregan, M., et al. "Milk Prolactin, Feed Volume and Duration Between Feeds in Women Breastfeeding Their Full Term Infants over a 24-Hour Period." *Experimental Physiology* 87 (2002): 207–214.

Daly, S., and P. Hartmann. "Infant Demand and Milk Supply. Part 2: The Short-Term Control of Milk Synthesis in Lactating Women." *Journal of Human Lactation* 11 (1995): 27–37.

Daly, S., et al. "Degree of Breast Emptying Explains Changes in the Fat Content, but Not Fatty Acid Composition, of Human Milk." *Experimental Physiology* 78 (1993): 741–755.

Dewey, K. "What Is the Optimal Age for Introduction of Complementary Foods?" *Nestle Nutrition Workshop Series* 58 (2006): 161–170.

Dewey, K., et al. "Risk Factors for Sub-Optimal Infant Breastfeeding Behavior, Delayed Onset of Lactation, and Excess Neonatal Weight Loss." *Pediatrics* 112 (2003): 607–619.

Diehl-Jones, W., and D. Askin. "Nutritional Modulation of Neonatal Outcomes." *AACN Clinical Issues Advanced Practice Acute Critical Care* 15 (2004): 83–96.

England, P., and R. Horowitz. *Birthing from Within*. Albuquerque: Partera Press, 1998.

Ersin, N., et al. "Association of Maternal-Child Characteristics as a Factor in Early Childhood Caries Salivary Bacterial Counts." *Journal of Dentistry for Children* 73 (2006): 105–111.

Freeman, M., et al. "Prolactin: Structure, Function, and Regulation of Secretion." *Physiological Reviews* 80 (2000): 8–31.

Fulhan, J., et al. "Update on Pediatric Nutrition: Breastfeeding, Infant Nutrition, and Growth." *Current Opinion in Pediatrics* 15 (2003): 323–332.

Gaskin, I. *Ina May's Guide to Guide to Childbirth*. New York: Bantam Books, 2003.

Graves, S., et al. "Painful Nipples in Nursing Mothers: Fungal or Staphylococcal?" *Australian Family Physician* 32 (2003): 570–571.

Gray, L., et al. "Breastfeeding Is Analgesic in Healthy Newborns." *Pediatrics* 109 (2002): 590–593.

Griffin, I., and S. Abrams. "Iron Metabolism in Human Milk–Fed Infants." *La Leche League International Study Module* 11 (2003): 4–19.

Hale, T. *Medications and Mothers' Milk,* 12th ed. Amarillo, TX: Hale Publishing, 2006.

Hartmann, P. "Initiation of Lactation in Term and Pre-Term Mothers." Lecture at 10th Annual Breastfeeding Conference; Baystate Health Systems Office of Continuing Education, 2005.

Heiser, B., and M. Walker. "Selling Out Mothers and Babies, Marketing of Breast Milk Substitutes." (2007); available from marsha@naba-breastfeeding.org.

Hoover, K. *The Link Between Infants' Oral Thrush and Nipple and Breast Pain in Lactating Women,* 4th ed. Mortan, PA: Self-Published Handout, 2001.

Hyams, J., et al. "Effect of Infant Formula on Stool Characteristics of Young Infants." *Pediatrics* 95 (1995): 50–54.

Jakobsson, I. "Food Antigens in Human Milk." *European Journal of Clinical Nutrition* 45 (1991): 29–33.

Johnson, R., ed. *Whole Foods for the Whole Family.* La Leche League International, 1993.

Keefe, M. "The Impact of Infant Rooming-In on Maternal Sleep at Night." *JOGNN* 17 (1988): 122–126.

Kenda, M. *Whole Foods for Babies and Toddlers.* La Leche League International, 2001.

Kendall-Tackett, K. *The Hidden Feelings of Motherhood,* 2nd ed. Amarillo, TX: Pharmasoft Publishing, 2005.

Kendall-Tackett, K. "Post-Partum Depression and the Breastfeeding Mother, Part I: Cause and Consequences." *La Leche League Independent Study Module* 5 (2003): 1–31.

Kennedy, K. "Premature Introduction of Progestin-Only Contraceptive Methods During Lactation." *Contraception* 55 (1997): 347–350.

Kulski, J., and P. Hartmann. "Changes in Human Milk Composition During the Initiation of Lactation." *The Australian Journal of Experimental Biology and Science* 59 (1981): 101–114.

Labbok, M., et al. "Multicenter Study of the Lactational Amenorrhea Method (LAM): I. Efficacy, Duration, and Implications for Clinical Application." *Contraception* 55 (1997): 327–336.

Lavender, T., et al. "Breastfeeding and Family Life." *Maternal and Child Nutrition* 2 (2006): 145–155.

Lewallen, L., et al. "Breastfeeding Support and Early Cessation." *JOGNN* 35 (2006): 166–172.

Ludington-Hoe, S., et al. "Infant Crying: Nature, Physiologic Consequences, and Select Intervention." *Neonatal Network* 21 (2002): 29–36.

Mangels, A., and V. Messina. "Considerations in Planning Vegan Diets: Infants." *Journal of the American Dietetic Association* 101 (2001): 670–677.

Massachusetts Breastfeeding Coalition. "What's Wrong with Those Cute Formula 'Gift' Bags?" (2006); www.massbfc.org.

Mennella, J. "Garlic Ingestion by Pregnant Women Alters the Odor of Amniotic Fluid." *Chemical Senses* 11 (1995): 39–45.

Mennella, J. "Mother's Milk: A Medium for Early Flavor Experiences." *Journal of Human Lactation* 11 (1995): 39–45.

Menella, J., and G. Beauchamp. "Mothers' Milk Enhances the Acceptance of Cereal During Weaning." *Pediatric Research* 41 (1997): 188–192.

Menella, J., and G. Beauchamp. "Maternal Diet Alters the Sensory Qualities of Human Milk and the Nursling's Behavior." *Pediatrics* 88 (1991): 737–744.

Mezzacappa, E., and E. Katkin. "Breastfeeding Is Associated with Reduced Perceived Stress and Negative Mood in Mothers." *Health Psychology* 21 (2002): 187–193.

Mitoulas, L., et al. "Variation in Fat, Lactose, and Protein in Human Milk Over 24h and Throughout the First Year of Lactation." *British Journal of Nutrition* 88 (2002): 29–37.

Mohrbacher, N., and K. Kendall-Tackett. *Breastfeeding Made Simple.* Oakland, CA: New Harbinger Publications, Inc., 2005.

Morrill, J., et al. "Risk Factors for Mammary Candidiasis Among Lactating Women." *JOGNN* 34 (2005): 37–45.

Neifert, M., et al. "Nipple Confusion: Toward a Formal Definition." *Journal of Pediatrics* 126 (1995): 125–129.

Panksepp, J. "Oxytocin Effects on Emotional Processes: Separation Distress, Social Bonding, and Relationships to Psychiatric Disorders." *Annals of the New York Academy of Sciences* 652 (1992): 243–252.

Pessl, M. "Exclusive Breastfeeding: Does It Matter?" Connecticut Breastfeeding Coalition Lecture Syllabus (2006): 1–8.

Queenan, J. T. "Contraception and Breastfeeding." *Clinical Obstetrics and Gynecology* 47 (2004): 734–739.

Quillin, S., and L. Glenn. "Interaction Between Feeding Method and Co-Sleeping on Maternal/Newborn Sleep." *JOGNN* 33 (2004): 580–588.

Ransjo-Arvidson, A., et al. "Maternal Analgesia During Labor Disturbs Newborn Behavior: Effects on Breastfeeding, Temperature, and Crying." *Birth* 28 (2001): 5–12.

Riordan, J. *Breastfeeding and Human Lactation,* 3rd ed. Sudbury, MA: Jones and Bartlett Publishers, 2005.

Riordan, J., et al. "The Effect of Labor Pain Relief Medication on Neonatal Suckling and Breastfeeding Duration." *Journal of Human Lactation* 16 (2000): 7–12.

Roepke, J. "Appropriate Introduction of Complementary Foods into the Diet of the Exclusively Breastfed Infant." *La Leche League International Study Module* 14 (2005): 1–16.

Souto, G., et al. "The Impact of Breast Reduction Surgery on Breastfeeding Performance." *Journal of Human Lactation* 19 (2003): 43–49.

Sowers, M., et al. "Changes in Bone Density with Lactation." *JAMA* 296 (1993): 3130–3135.

Swanson, V., and K. G. Power. "Initiation and Continuation of Breastfeeding: Theory of Planned Behavior." *Journal of Advanced Nursing* 50 (2004): 272–282.

Tanguay, K., et al. "Nipple Candidiasis Among Breastfeeding Mothers." *Canadian Family Physician* 40 (1994): 1407–1413.

Truitt, S. T., et al. "Combined Hormonal Versus Nonhormonal Versus Progestin Only Contraception in Lactation." *The Cochrane Collaboration* 1 (2007): 1–14.

Vidaeff, A. "Breech Delivery Before and After Term Breech Trial." *Clinical Obstetrics* 49 (2006): 198–210.

Walker, M. *Core Curriculum for Lactation Consultant Practice.* Sudbury, MA: Jones and Bartlett Publishers, 2002.

Walker, M. "Do Labor Medications Affect Breastfeeding?" *Journal of Human Lactation* 13 (1997): 131–137.

Walker, M. "Just One Bottle Won't Hurt—Or Will It?" *Supplementation of the Breastfed Baby* (2007); www.massbfc.org/formula/bottle.html.

Walker, M. "Mastitis in Lactating Women." *La Leche League International Study Module* 6 (2004): 1–19.

Whiffen, V., and I. Gotlib. "Infants of Post-Partum Depressed Mothers; Temperament and Cognitive Status." *Journal of Abnormal Psychology* 98 (1989): 274–279.

Wilumsen, J., et al. "Breastmilk RNA Viral Load in HIV-Infected South African Women: Effects of Sub-Clinical Mastitis and Infant Feeding." *AIDS* 17 (2003): 407–414.

Winberg, J. "Mother and Newborn Baby: Mutual Regulation of Physiology and Behavior—A Selective Review." *Developmental Psychobiology* 47 (2005): 217–229.

World Health Organization. "Global Strategy for Infant and Young Child Feeding." World Health Organization Geneva (2003): 7–8.

Zinaman, M., et al. "Acute Prolactin and Oxytocin Responses and Milk Yield to Infant Suckling and Artificial Methods of Expression in Lactating Women." *Pediatrics* 89 (1992) 437–440.

Index